A T L A S O F

NEUROLOGIC
DIAGNOSIS AND TREATMENT

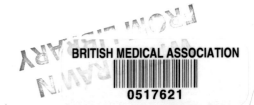

ATLAS OF
NEUROLOGIC
DIAGNOSIS AND TREATMENT

R. DOUGLAS COLLINS, MD, FACP
Neurology and Internal Medicine
Bonifay, Florida

WENDY BETH JACKELOW
Medical and Scientific Illustration

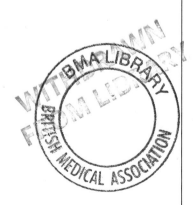

LIPPINCOTT WILLIAMS & WILKINS
A **Wolters Kluwer** Company

Philadelphia · Baltimore · New York · London
Buenos Aires · Hong Kong · Sydney · Tokyo

Acquisitions Editor: Danette Somers
Editorial Coordinator: Mary Choi
Project Manager: Nicole Walz
Senior Manufacturing Manager: Ben Rivera
Senior Marketing Manager: Kathy Neely
Creative Director: Doug Smock
Cover Designer: Joseph De Pinho
Compositor: MD Composition, Inc.
Printer: Edwards Brothers

Printed in the United States of America

Library of Congress Cataloging-in-Publication Data

Collins, R. Douglas.
  Atlas of neurologic diagnosis and treatment / R. Douglas Collins. -- 1st ed.
    p. ; cm.
  Includes bibliographical references and index.
  ISBN 0-7817-9511-7
  1. Nervous system--Diseases--Handbooks, manuals, etc. 2. Nervous system--Diseases--Atlases. 3. Diagnosis, Differential.
4. Primary care (Medicine) I. Title.
  [DNLM: 1. Diagnostic Techniques, Neurological--Atlases. 2. Nervous system Diseases--therapy--Atlases. WL 17 C712a 2004]
RC355.C64 2004
616.8'0022'2—dc22

                                        2004015192

To purchase additional copies of this book, call our customer service department at **(800) 638-3030** or fax orders to **(301) 824-7390.** International customers should call **(301) 714-2324.**

Visit Lippincott Williams & Wilkins on the Internet: http://www.LWW.com. Lippincott Williams & Wilkins customer service representatives are available from 8:30 am to 6:00 pm, EST.

05 06 07 08 09
1 2 3 4 5 6 7 8 9 10

To my grandchildren, Oliver, Peyton, Cathleen, Jahrel, Jeron, Alex, Brandon, and Azsalyn.

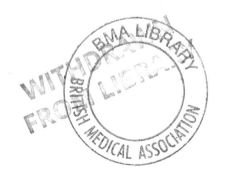

PREFACE

Neurology is undoubtedly the most complex subject facing medical students and clinicians. It involves the study of literally thousands of diseases and syndromes involving a maze of neuroanatomical structures. Consequently, physicians are tempted to refer the patient with neurologic symptoms to a neurologic specialist or to order an expensive diagnostic test such as a CT scan or MRI.

There is a need for a book that will simplify neurology and make it possible for the primary care clinicians to diagnose and treat patients with neurologic conditions—a book that will heighten the awareness of non-neurologic specialists to these diseases. *Atlas of Neurologic Diagnosis and Treatment* is aimed at fulfilling this need.

In order to achieve this goal, the author has adhered to the following principles:

1. Diseases are colorfully illustrated on easy to understand neuroanatomical drawings.
2. Diseases are brought to life by case reports picturing the salient features of each disease.
3. A synopsis of etiology, diagnosis and treatment accompanies each report.
4. The differential diagnosis of neurologic symptoms and signs is addressed and arranged in alphabetical order for easy reference.
5. Diagnostic tests that may be ordered for each disease are listed in Appendix B.
6. Treatment of each disease is addressed in Appendix C for easy reference.
7. Rare diseases, controversial diagnostic procedures, and treatment are omitted, but the reader is referred to excellent references for further study of these subjects.

It is the hope of the author that this text will promote a more widespread interest and clinical application of neurologic diagnosis and treatment.

Many individuals have helped in the development of the project but only a few will be mentioned here. Wendy Beth Jackelow took my primitive sketches and turned them into the beautiful neuroanatomical illustrations in this book. My wife, Norie, spent countless hours typing the manuscript, and my daughter, L. Joy, transferred it to a computer disc for submission to the publisher.

Finally, I want to thank Danette Somers and the staff at Lippincott Williams & Wilkins for their assistance in making my dreams a reality.

R. DOUGLAS COLLINS, MD, FACP

TABLE OF CONTENTS

Part Two

The Differential Diagnosis of Neurologic Signs   49

The Routine Neurologic Examination   49

Part Three

Diseases of the Spinal Cord, Peripheral Nerves, and Muscles *83*

Part Four

Diseases of the Brain and Brainstem   *121*

PART ONE

The Differential Diagnosis of Neurologic Symptoms

The Neurologic History

By the time you picked up this book, you probably had already developed your own method of history taking. Nevertheless, the following discussion may give you a few useful tips to apply in this important process.

Rather than taking the patient's history in a robotic way, it is important to approach him or her with a list of diagnostic possibilities based on his or her chief complaint. We often form this list of possibilities by a sense of what the common diagnosis is for the particular chief complaint. For example, if a patient complains of headache, the diagnoses of migraine, hypertensive, and muscle contraction headaches might quickly come to mind. However, wouldn't it be better to have a more complete list of possibilities in mind as we approach this patient? To do that, I use the mnemonic *VINDICATE*: *V* for *vascular*, *I* for *inflammatory*, *N* for *neoplastic*, *D* for degenerative, *I* for *intoxication*, *C* for *congenital*, *A* for *autoimmune*, *T* for *trauma*, and *E* for *endocrine*.

Applying this mnemonic to the chief complaint of headache, *vascular* brings to mind migraine, histamine cephalgia, and temporal arteritis; *inflammation* indicates meningitis, encephalitis, and cerebral abscess; *neoplastic* suggests brain tumor; *degenerative* brings to mind cervical spondylosis and degenerative disc disease; *intoxication* prompts consideration of drug-induced or caffeine-withdrawal headaches; *congenital* points to cerebral aneurysms and subarachnoid hemorrhage; *autoimmune* indicates lupus and concussion; *trauma* suggests epidural or subdural hematoma and concussion; and *endocrine* prompts consideration of pheochromocytoma.

The mnemonic process allows us to develop the chief complaint in a more meaningful way. Further development of the chief complaint may be made by considering the mode of onset, severity, duration, and frequency of the symptom(s), as well as associated symptoms.

Onset: An acute onset suggests a traumatic, toxic, vascular, or inflammatory etiology, whereas a gradual onset suggests a neoplastic or degenerative process. Exceptions to this rule are abscess; neurosyphilis, which may have a gradual onset; and metastatic neoplasm, which may have an acute onset.

Severity: The severity of a symptom ought to correlate with the seriousness of the diagnosis, but that is frequently not the case. For example, migraine headaches are severe, whereas headaches due to brain tumor are often mild. However, serious conditions such as bacterial meningitis and subarachnoid hemorrhage are associated with severe headaches.

Duration: The duration of a complaint assists in the diagnosis. For example, migraine headaches last hours to days, cluster headaches last minutes to hours, attacks of trigeminal neuralgia typically last seconds, and the headaches of a space-occupying lesion are almost continuous. Again, petit mal seizures last seconds whereas complex partial seizures and grand mal seizures usually last several minutes.

Frequency: The frequency of attacks is a key to the diagnosis. Muscle contraction headaches may be continuous, whereas cluster headaches recur daily. The headaches of meningitis and temporal arteritis are continuous until therapeutic intervention is obtained.

Associated Symptoms: It is rare for a patient to present with one isolated symptom. For example, if the patient has pain, there may be a lump in the painful area. If the patient has an earache, there may be a discharge associated with it. If the patient presents with a headache, does he or she have nausea and/or vomiting? If the answer is yes, consider migraine or a space-occupying lesion at the top of your list. For a more organized approach, associated symptoms may be grouped into several categories: pain, lump or mass, bloody discharge, nonbloody discharge, and functional changes. It is the combination of symptoms that often nails down the diagnosis. For example, a right-sided headache with a large and tender temporal artery would suggest temporal arteritis, whereas a headache with blurred vision may suggest glaucoma.

Review of Systems

The traditional review of systems is boring and time consuming. I find it easier and more focused to use the same technique applied with associated symptoms in the review of systems. Thus, I take the categories of pain, lump or mass, bloody discharge, nonbloody discharge, and functional changes, and apply them to the systems. Using this method, I question the patient as follows:

Pain: Do you have any pain in your head, eyes, ears, mouth, neck, chest, abdomen, or extremities? Is there pain on swallowing, breathing, defecating, or urinating?

Lump or Mass: Have you noticed a lump or mass in your head, neck, chest, abdomen, back, bottom, or extremities?

Bloody Discharge: Have you had bleeding from your nose or ears? Have you coughed up or vomited blood, or had blood in your urine or stool or under your skin?

Nonbloody Discharge: Have you experienced a discharge from your eyes, ears, nose, or throat? Have you had a chronic productive cough or rectal, urethral, or vaginal discharge?

Functional Changes: Have you had visual loss or disturbances, hearing loss, ringing in your ears, dizziness, cough, shortness of breath, nausea or vomiting, palpitations, loss of appetite, hunger, diarrhea, constipation, frequency of urination, difficulty voiding, loss of libido, disturbances of menstruation, difficulty walking, etc.?

Past History: Here you can simply ask if the patient has had heart disease, lung disease, liver disease, stomach or intestinal disease, kidney disease, rectal disease, or diseases of reproductive organs. Also ask the patient if he or she ever had surgery on any of these organs.

Family History: This is important to the neurologic history as many diseases are hereditary. Not only should you ask whether there has been a specific neurologic disease in the family, but you should also ask general questions such as: Did your mom or dad have difficulty walking, tremor, trouble with vision, dizziness, etc.?

I hope this discussion makes your history taking more dynamic and enjoyable. Now, turning to each symptom is this section, you will find additional questions you may ask your patients to help you pin down the diagnosis.

AMNESIA

In the history, is there:
1. **Recent head trauma?** Consider concussion or subdural or epidural hematoma.
2. **Alcohol abuse?** Consider alcohol blackouts, Wernicke's encephalopathy, or Korsakoff syndrome.
3. **Atherosclerotic disease?** Consider cerebral ischemia or transient global ischemia.
4. **Systemic cancer?** Consider paraneoplastic limbic encephalitis.
5. **Recent viral encephalitis?** Consider postencephalitic amnesia, particularly associated with herpes simplex virus.
6. **Anxiety or depression?** Consider dissociative or psychogenic amnesia.
7. **Migraine?** Consider transient global amnesia due to migraine.
8. **Epilepsy?** Consider fugue state of temporal lobe epilepsy.

On physical examination, is (are) there:
1. **Papilledema or focal neurologic signs?** Consider brain tumor or cerebrovascular disease.
2. **Unilateral or bilateral hemianopsia?** Consider unilateral or bilateral posterior cerebral artery occlusion.
3. **Ophthalmoplegia?** Consider Wernicke's encephalopathy.

Diagnostic Workup
1. Drug screen (drug intoxication)
2. Blood alcohol level (alcoholism, Wernicke's encephalopathy)
3. MRI (brain tumor, hematoma)
4. EEG (epilepsy, drug intoxication)
5. Spinal tap (encephalitis)
6. Psychometric testing (psychogenic amnesia)
7. Neurologic consultation
8. Psychiatric consultation

ANOSMIA OR UNUSUAL ODOR

Anosmia is loss of the sense of smell. The lesion is usually in the nose or olfactory bulb or tract.

In the history, is (are) there:
1. **Symptoms of nasal congestion or cough?** Consider acute upper respiratory infection, acute or chronic rhinitis or sinusitis, or hay fever.
2. **Head trauma?** Consider concussion or fracture of the cribriform plate.
3. **Drug use?** Cocaine and prolonged use of nasal decongestants are well-recognized causes of anosmia, but amphetamines, phenothiazine, or estrogen may also be the cause.
4. **Exposure to lead?** Lead poisoning may cause anosmia.
5. **Diabetes mellitus?** This condition is known to cause anosmia.
6. **Intermittent anosmia or unusual odors?** This would prompt consideration of temporal lobe epilepsy.
7. **Anxiety, depression, or other emotional disturbance?** Consider a psychiatric disorder.

On physical examination, is (are) there:
1. **Papilledema?** Think of olfactory groove meningioma or other space-occupying lesion.
2. **Nasal discharge?** Think of rhinitis, sinusitis, neoplasm, or midline granuloma.
3. **Hemiparesis or other focal neurologic signs?** Consider brain tumor, abscess or hematoma, or cerebral embolism or thrombosis.
4. **Signs of systemic disease?** Consider hypothyroidism, cirrhosis, renal failure, or pernicious anemia.
5. **Unilateral anosmia?** Consider possible olfactory groove meningioma.

Diagnostic Workup
1. Complete blood count (upper respiratory infection, sinusitis, pernicious anemia)
2. Urine screen (drug abuse)
3. Blood lead level
4. Radiograph of the sinuses (sinusitis)
5. Culture of nasal discharge (sinusitis, rhinitis)
6. CT scan (skull fracture, brain tumor)
7. Chemistry panel (diabetes, cirrhosis, renal failure)
8. EEG (temporal lobe epilepsy)
9. Psychiatric consultation (psychiatric disorder)

ANXIETY

In the history, is (are) there:
1. **Evidence that the anxiety is intermittent?** Consider epilepsy, pheochromocytoma, or insulinoma.
2. **Associated polyuria, polyphagia, and weight loss?** Consider hyperthyroidism.
3. **Head trauma?** Consider postconcussion syndrome.
4. **Drug use or abuse?** Consider drug side effects or withdrawal symptoms.
5. **Alcohol, cigarette, or caffeine use?** These are common causes of chronic anxiety.
6. **Senility?** Consider various forms of dementia (see page 33).
7. **Emotional problems?** Consider psychiatric disorder.

On physical examination, is (are) there:
1. **Tachycardia?** Consider hyperthyroidism, pheochromocytoma, cardiac arrhythmia, or caffeine or drug use.
2. **Tremor and chronic diaphoresis?** Consider hyperthyroidism, nicotine, and caffeine in the differential diagnosis.

Diagnostic Workup
1. Complete blood count
2. Urinalysis
3. Chemistry panel
4. Urine drug screen (alcohol and drug abuse)
5. Free thyroxine (hyperthyroidism)
6. 24-hour vanillylmandelic acid or catecholamines (pheochromocytoma)
7. EKG (cardiac arrhythmia)
8. EEG (epilepsy)
9. Psychiatric consultation (chronic anxiety, neurosis)
10. Psychometric testing (psychiatric disorder)

BACK PAIN

Back pain may be focal or diffuse. The lesion is usually in the spine but may be found in the visceral organs or the meninges.

In the history, is there:

1. **Acute onset?** Acute onset of back pain is associated with sprain, herniated disc, epidural abscess, and fractures of the spine. However, abdominal conditions such as renal colic, pyelonephritis, ruptured peptic ulcer, pancreatitis, or dissecting aneurysm may present with an acute onset. Gradual onset of back pain is associated with metastatic or primary neoplasms of the spine and spinal cord and rheumatoid spondylitis. Congenital anomalies of the spine, such as scoliosis, may present with a gradual onset of back pain. Abdominal conditions such as pancreatic carcinoma and endometriosis may present with a gradual onset of back pain.
2. **Recent trauma?** This would prompt consideration of sprains, herniated disc, and fractures of the spine. Trauma may also precipitate or exacerbate spondylolisthesis and other congenital anomalies. Lumbar spondylosis may be silent until a traumatic event.
3. **Fever?** Consider epidural abscess, osteomyelitis of the spine, pyelonephritis, or an infectious disease such as dengue fever, undulant fever, or tuberculosis.
4. **Radiation of pain around the trunk or into the extremities?** Consider osteoarthritis, rheumatoid spondylitis, or sprains.
5. **Frequency of urination or difficulty voiding?** Consider space-occupying lesion of the spinal cord, such as neoplasm, abscess, or hematoma. Also, consider kidney disease in all or pelvic conditions in women.
6. **Anxiety or depression?** Consider hysteria, hypochondriasis, or malingering.

On physical examination, is (are) there:

1. **A positive straight leg–raising test or femoral stretch test?** Consider a herniated disc or other cause of radiculopathy.
2. **Focal neurologic signs?** Consider herniated disc or other space-occupying lesion of the spinal cord or nerve roots.
3. **Hematuria?** Consider renal calculus, neoplasm, or urinary tract infection.
4. **Pelvic mass?** Consider ovarian tumor, uterine tumor, pelvic inflammatory disease, or endometriosis.
5. **Prostatic mass?** Consider carcinoma of the prostate with metastasis or prostatitis.

Diagnostic Workup

1. Complete blood count, urinalysis, urine culture (pyelonephritis, renal colic)
2. Chemistry panel (metastatic neoplasm)
3. Serum protein electrophoresis (multiple myeloma)
4. Human leukocyte antigen B27 (rheumatoid spondylitis)
5. MRI or CT scan of the spine (herniated disc, spinal cord tumor abscess, or hematoma)
6. Bone scan (metastatic tumor, osteomyelitis, rheumatoid spondylitis)
7. CT scan of abdomen and pelvis (abdominal or pelvic neoplasm)
8. Neurologic consultation (tumor, disc)
9. Gynecologic consultation (pelvic mass)
10. Psychiatric consultation (neurosis, malingering)

BLINDNESS

Blindness may be bilateral or unilateral. The lesion may be anywhere between the eye and the brain.

In the history, is there:
1. **Intermittent blindness?** Consider transient ischemic attacks, epilepsy, or migraine.
2. **Acute onset?** Acute onset of blindness occurs in carotid artery thrombosis, posterior cerebral artery thrombosis or embolism, temporal arteritis, optic neuritis, retinal vein thrombosis, retinal artery thrombosis, detached retina, multiple sclerosis, and hysteria. Gradual onset of blindness is consistent with glaucoma, uveitis, retinitis, brain tumors, and tumors of the optic nerves.
3. **Monocular blindness?** Consider vitreous hemorrhage, optic neuritis, retinal vein thrombosis, retinal artery occlusion, optic nerve injuries, detached retina, fracture of the skull, retinoblastoma, or sphenoid ridge meningioma. If the blindness is bilateral, consider a cerebral artery occlusion, muscular degeneration, hereditary optic atrophy, cataracts, multiple sclerosis, iritis, glaucoma, or toxic amblyopia.
4. **Headache?** Consider migraine, glaucoma, or space-occupying lesions of the brain.

On physical examination, is (are) there:
1. **Papilledema?** Consider optic neuritis, retinal vein thrombosis, or space-occupying lesions of the brain.
2. **Optic atrophy?** Consider hereditary optic atrophy, pituitary adenoma or other brain tumors compressing the optic nerve, toxic amblyopia, or glaucoma.
3. **Increased intraocular pressure?** Consider glaucoma.
4. **Focal neurologic signs in the extremities?** Consider brain tumor, multiple sclerosis, or cerebrovascular disease.
5. **Other abnormalities on ophthalmoscopic examination?** Ophthalmoscopic examination may show cataracts, iritis, retinitis pigmentosus, detached retina, vitreous hemorrhages, the pale retina and cherry-red spot of retinal artery occlusion, or retinoblastoma.

Diagnostic Workup
1. Ophthalmologic consultation
2. Slit lamp examination (uveitis)
3. Tonometry (glaucoma)
4. Visual field examination (pituitary neoplasm, optic neuritis)
5. Neurologic consultation
6. Carotid duplex scan (carotid artery occlusion or stenosis)
7. MRI or CT scan (space-occupying lesion, multiple sclerosis, cerebrovascular disease)
8. Four-vessel cerebral angiography (cerebrovascular disease, aneurysms)
9. EEG (hysterical blindness, malingering)

BLURRED VISION

The lesion is usually in the eye or optic nerve but may be in the brain or brainstem.

In the history, is (are) there:
1. **Recent head trauma?** Consider corneal abrasions, retinal detachment, concussion, or subdural hematoma.
2. **Acute onset?** This should prompt consideration of migraine, optic neuritis, vitreous hemorrhage, retinal artery occlusion, glaucoma, iritis, keratitis, retinal detachment, carotid artery thrombosis, orbital fracture, or hysteria.
3. **Intermittent episodes?** Consider migraine, carotid artery insufficiency, or epilepsy.
4. **Only one eye involved?** Consider local ocular conditions such as glaucoma, keratitis, foreign body, iritis, optic neuritis, or retinal detachment. Bilateral blurred vision aside from refraction errors and astigmatism is more likely a result of systemic causes. In that case, consider methyl alcohol poisoning, barbiturate intoxication, quinine, cocaine, or other drugs. Also consider febrile conditions, concussion, migraine, or hysteria. Local conditions mentioned above must also be considered when there is bilateral blurred vision.
5. **Headache or eye pain?** Consider migraine, glaucoma, foreign body, or space-occupying lesions of the brain.
6. **A history of drug use or abuse?** Consider cocaine, heroin, tobacco, quinine, barbiturate, or methyl alcohol use.

On physical examination, is (are) there:
1. **Ocular discharge?** Consider keratitis, conjunctivitis, corneal abrasions, foreign body, or lacrimal duct obstruction.
2. **Corneal or lens opacities?** Consider keratitis or cataracts.
3. **Elevated intraocular pressure?** Consider glaucoma.
4. **Focal neurologic signs in the other cranial nerves or extremities?** Consider space-occupying lesions of the brain, cerebrovascular disease, or multiple sclerosis.
5. **Visual field abnormalities?** Consider optic neuritis, multiple sclerosis, pituitary adenoma, or other brain tumor. Also consider cerebrovascular disease.

Diagnostic Workup
1. Toxicology screen
2. Ophthalmologic consultation
3. Slit lamp examination (keratitis)
4. Tonometry (glaucoma)
5. Visual fields (optic neuritis, brain tumor)
6. Neurologic consultation
7. Carotid ultrasonography (carotid insufficiency)
8. Sedimentation rate (temporal arteritis)
9. CT scan or MRI (space-occupying lesion)
10. Spinal tap (multiple sclerosis, neurosyphilis)
11. Four-vessel cerebral angiography (cerebrovascular disease)

COMA

Coma is a loss of consciousness. The lesion is usually in the brain or brainstem but may be psychogenic.

In the history, is there:
1. **Trauma?** Consider concussion, epidural or subdural hematoma, skull fracture, or intracerebral hemorrhage.
2. **Diabetes?** Consider diabetic coma, hyperosmolar coma, or insulin shock.
3. **Epilepsy?** Consider status epilepticus, concussion or subdural hematoma.
4. **Alcohol use?** Consider severe alcohol intoxication, Wernicke's encephalopathy, or subdural hematoma.
5. **Drug use?** Consider drug intoxication.
6. **Upper respiratory or other systemic infection?** Consider meningitis or brain abscess.
7. **Liver or kidney disease?** Consider hepatic or renal failure.
8. **Cardiac disease?** Consider cerebral embolism or subacute bacterial endocarditis (SBE).
9. **Psychiatric disorder?** Consider suicide attempt or drug reaction.

On physical examination, is (are) there:
1. **Ecchymosis or evidence of fractures?** Consider concussion or epidural or subdural hematoma.
2. **Nuchal rigidity?** Consider subarachnoid hemorrhage or meningitis.
3. **Unusual odor to breath?** Consider diabetic coma, alcohol intoxication, hepatic coma, uremia, etc.
4. **Dilated pupil(s)?** A unilateral dilated pupil suggests a space-occupying lesion such as a subdural hematoma. Bilateral dilated pupils may indicate drug intoxication.
5. **Constricted pupils?** Constricted pupils may indicate morphine or other drug intoxication as well as a pontine hemorrhage.
6. **Hemiparesis or other focal neurologic signs?** Consider stroke or space-occupying lesions of the brain.
7. **Retinal hemorrhages?** Consider diabetic coma, subarachnoid hemorrhage, SBE, or collagen disease.
8. **Papilledema?** Consider space-occupying lesion of the brain, malignant hypertension, or other causes of increased intracranial pressure.
9. **Lacerated tongue?** Consider epilepsy.
10. **Cherry-red lips?** Consider carbon monoxide poisoning.
11. **Needle tracks?** Consider heroin addiction.
12. **Heart murmur or arrhythmia?** Consider cerebral embolism or SBE.
13. **Petechial hemorrhages?** Consider meningococcal meningitis, SBE, or blood dyscrasias.
14. **Resistance to eye opening?** Consider hysteria.

Diagnostic Workup
1. Immediate complete blood count and chemistry panel (diabetes, infectious disease, hepatic or renal failure)
2. Response to intravenous dextrose and thiamine (insulin shock, Wernicke's encephalopathy)
3. Urine drug screen (drug intoxication)
4. Blood alcohol level
5. Blood ammonia (liver failure)
6. Arterial blood gas analysis (respiratory failure, shock)
7. Neurologic consultation
8. Radiography of the skull and cervical spine (fracture, hematoma)
9. CT scan (brain tumor or subdural or epidural hematoma)
10. Spinal tap (meningitis, subarachnoid hemorrhage)
11. EEG (status epilepticus, drug intoxication)
12. Cardiologic consultation (cerebral embolism)

CONVULSIONS

Convulsions are involuntary tonic or clonic movements of the face or extremities usually associated with loss of consciousness. They may be focal or diffuse. The lesion is in the cerebrum.

In the history, is (are) there:
1. **Evidence of recent or past head injury?** This would suggest the possibility of an epidural, subdural, or intracerebral hematoma. Even a tiny unresolved hematoma may cause scarring and become an epileptogenic focus.
2. **Drug use or abuse?** Withdrawal seizures may occur from many drugs, including barbiturates and benzodiazepines. Seizures may result from the use of phenothiazine. Many drugs may cause seizures when abused, most noticeably cocaine, heroin, and amphetamines.
3. **A family history of convulsions?** Consider lipid storage disease, porphyria, or phenylketonuria, among other hereditary disorders.
4. **Fever and chills?** Seizures may be caused by infectious diseases such as viral encephalitis, bacterial meningitis, syphilis, tuberculosis, brain abscess, human immunodeficiency virus (HIV), and malaria and other parasites. Febrile convulsions should be considered in children.
5. **Evidence of birth defects, trauma, or anoxia?** Look for Down syndrome, toxoplasmosis, Tay-Sachs disease, tuberous sclerosis, or Sturge-Weber disease. If the delivery was difficult, consider birth trauma or anoxia. Kernicterus from erythroblastosis fetalis may cause seizures.
6. **Seizures without an aura, incontinence of urine, tongue lacerations, or postictal phenomena?** Consider psychogenic epilepsy.
7. **Evidence of focal or jacksonian-type convulsions?** Consider a space-occupying lesion.

In the physical examination, is (are) there:
1. **Papilledema?** Consider a brain tumor, hematoma, or abscess.
2. **Focal neurologic signs?** Consider a space-occupying lesion or cerebrovascular disease.
3. **Nuchal rigidity?** Consider meningitis or subarachnoid hemorrhage.
4. **Unusual odor to breath?** Consider alcohol intoxication or withdrawal, diabetic coma, hepatic failure, or uremia.
5. **Rash?** Consider tuberous sclerosis, Sturge-Weber disease, neurofibromatosis, collagen disease, or subacute bacterial endocarditis.
6. **Cardiac arrhythmia or murmur?** Look for cerebral embolism.
7. **Enlarged liver or spleen?** Consider alcoholism, hepatic failure, collagen disease, or blood dyscrasias.

Diagnostic Workup
1. Complete blood count
2. Chemistry panel (diabetes, uremia, hypoglycemia)
3. Antinuclear antibody activity (collagen disease)
4. Venereal Disease Research Laboratory (VDRL) test (neurosyphilis)
5. EEG, awake and asleep (symptomatic and idiopathic epilepsy)
6. Urine drug screen (drug and alcohol intoxication)
7. MRI (space-occupying lesion)
8. HIV testing (acquired immunodeficiency syndrome)
9. Spinal tap (meningitis, brain abscess, neurosyphilis, multiple sclerosis)
10. Ambulatory or hospital continuous EEG monitoring (idiopathic epilepsy, psychogenic epilepsy)
11. Visual evoked potential (multiple sclerosis)
12. Neurologic consultation (space-occupying lesion, stroke)

Treatment
Grand mal seizures are treated initially with valproate, phenytoin, or carbamazepine (see Appendix C for dosage and treatment schedules). It is important to try one drug at a time before using combination therapy. Occasionally, phenobarbital and primidone are useful either alone or in combination with other drugs; however, they are highly sedative. A neurologist should be consulted before using combination therapy or trying a newer antiepileptic drug, such as gabapentin, lamotrigine, or topiramate. All patients require initial and repeated hemograms and blood chemistries to catch bone marrow suppression and liver toxicity early. It is wise to monitor anticonvulsant blood levels frequently to regulate dosage and assure compliance.

Absence attacks may be prevented with valproate or ethosuximide. In some patients with combined grand mal and absence attacks, valproate may be used alone. Other patients respond to a combination of ethosuximide and phenytoin.

For most neurologists, the drug of choice for complex partial seizures is still carbamazepine. A neurologist should be consulted before one attempts different therapeutic combinations and dosages.

Status epilepticus is a life-threatening emergency that also requires a neurologist's attention. If a neurologist is not available, provide a good airway and cardiovascular support and give lorazepam, 4 mg intravenously over 2 minutes. This dosage may be repeated once in 10 minutes if seizures continue. If status continues, try fosphenytoin, 20 mg/kg intravenously at 150 mg/minute, with careful blood pressure and EEG monitoring. If status persists, give an additional 5 mg/kg of fosphenytoin two times for a total of 30 mg/kg. By this time, it is hoped that a neurologist is on the scene to supervise management.

DEAFNESS

Deafness is a loss of hearing. The lesion may be in the external, middle, or inner ear; the auditory nerve; or the brainstem.

In the history, is (are) there:
  1. **Sudden onset?** This would suggest a middle ear infection, trauma, or stroke. A gradual onset suggests neoplasm, drug intoxication, or degenerative process such as presbycusis or otosclerosis.
  2. **Only one ear involved?** Consider otitis media, acoustic neuroma, foreign body, trauma, or Meniere's disease. Bilateral involvement is more likely a result of otosclerosis, acoustic trauma, drug toxicity, or presbycusis.
  3. **Otalgia?** Pain in the ear is most likely a result of an infectious process or trauma. Painless deafness is more likely to be caused by a toxic, neoplastic, or degenerative process.
  4. **Ear discharge?** Obviously, this would prompt the consideration of otitis externa or media, foreign body, or local trauma. Cerebrospinal otorrhea should also be considered.
  5. **Fever?** Here again, one should consider an infectious process such as otitis media.
  6. **Drug exposure?** Gentamicin and other aminoglycosides are notorious for causing deafness, but quinine, salicylates, and furosemide should also be considered.
  7. **Headache?** Consider acoustic neuroma or other space-occupying lesion.
  8. **Vertigo?** Consider Meniere's disease, acoustic neuroma, multiple sclerosis, or basilar artery occlusion or insufficiency.
  9. **Weakness or paresthesias in the extremities?** Consider multiple sclerosis, brainstem tumor, or basilar artery insufficiency.
 10. **Intermittent deafness?** Suspect multiple sclerosis, Meniere's disease, or epilepsy.

On physical examination, is (are) there:
  1. **Abnormalities on otoscopic examination?** Consider otitis media or externa, foreign body, wax, or cholesteatoma.
  2. **Papilledema?** Consider a space-occupying lesion such as advanced acoustic neuroma.
  3. **Focal neurologic signs?** Consider multiple sclerosis, cerebrovascular disease, or acoustic neuroma.
  4. **Abnormal Weber or Rinne test?** The Weber test is helpful in establishing a diagnosis in unilateral deafness. If sound lateralizes to the normal ear, consider sensorineural deafness caused by acoustic neuroma, Meniere's disease, multiple sclerosis, or cholesteatoma. If it lateralizes to the affected ear, consider otitis media or otosclerosis. In the Rinne test, 2:1 air-to-bone conduction bilaterally indicates normal hearing. In otosclerosis and other cases of conductive deafness, the ratio is closer to 1:1. In sensorineural deafness, the conduction ratio remains 2:1 air to bone bilaterally or on the affected side.
  5. **Nystagmus?** Consider acoustic neuroma, Meniere's disease, or brainstem or cerebellar disease.
  6. **Nonpitting edema?** Consider hypothyroidism.

Diagnostic Workup
  1. Audiometry
  2. Caloric testing
  3. Electronystagmography (acoustic neuroma, Meniere's disease)
  4. Tympanography (otitis media)
  5. Otolaryngologic consultation
  6. MRI (space-occupying lesions, stroke, multiple sclerosis)
  7. Magnetic resonance angiography (basilar artery insufficiency or aneurysm)
  8. Brainstem evoked potentials (multiple sclerosis)
  9. Fluorescent treponemal absorption of blood and spinal fluid (neurosyphilis)
 10. Thyroid function studies (hypothyroidism)

DELIRIUM

Delirium is a slight to moderate depression of cerebral function with retention of consciousness but poor recognition of the environment and poor control of behavior. The lesion is psychogenic or cerebral.

In the history, is there:
1. **Recent trauma?** Consider concussion or epidural or subdural hematoma.
2. **Drug or alcohol abuse?** Consider drug toxicity or withdrawal, delirium tremens, or other syndromes caused by alcohol.
3. **Fever?** Consider meningitis, encephalitis, cerebral abscess, or hemorrhage.
4. **Exposure to toxic substances in the workplace?** Consider manganese, lead, or other substance.
5. **Diabetes?** Consider diabetic acidosis or hypoglycemia.

On physical examination, is (are) there:
1. **Nuchal rigidity?** Consider meningitis or subarachnoid hemorrhage.
2. **Papilledema?** Consider a space-occupying lesion of the brain.
3. **Focal neurologic signs?** Consider a space-occupying lesion.
4. **A sweet odor to the breath?** Consider diabetic acidosis or alcoholism.
5. **An unusual odor to the breath?** Consider uremia or hepatic failure.

Diagnostic Workup
1. Complete blood count (internal hemorrhage)
2. Chemistry panel (uremia, hepatic failure, diabetes, electrolyte disorder)
3. Blood cultures (septicemia or other bacteria infection)
4. Urine drug screen (Alcohol or drug toxicity)
5. Neurologic consultation
6. CT scan (hemorrhage, space-occupying lesion)
7. Spinal tap (meningitis, subarachnoid hemorrhage)
8. Response to intravenous thiamine (Wernicke's encephalopathy)
9. Response to intravenous glucose (hypoglycemia)
10. Arterial blood gases (respiratory failure)
11. Carboxyhemoglobin (carbon monoxide poisoning)
12. EEG (drug toxicity)
13. Urine porphobilinogen (porphyria)

DELUSIONS

Delusions are feelings or beliefs that have no reasonable explanation. They are almost always psychogenic but may be caused by an organic brain syndrome.

In the history, is (are) there:
1. **Drug or alcohol use?** Some drugs are associated with delusions, most notably cocaine, phencyclidine hydrochloride (PCP), and lysergic acid diethylamide (LSD). Alcoholics with Korsakoff syndrome may exhibit confabulation, thus simulating a delusional state.
2. **Possible venereal disease?** Consider the paranoid delusions of general paresis.
3. **Evidence of dementia?** Consider Alzheimer's disease or cerebral arteriosclerosis.
4. **Hallucinations or disturbances of affect?** Consider schizophrenia or manic-depressive psychosis.
5. **Depression?** Consider neurotic or psychotic depressive states.

Diagnostic Workup
1. Urine drug screen (drug or alcohol intoxication)
2. Fluorescent treponemal absorption of blood and spinal fluid (neurosyphilis)
3. Serum cortisol (Cushing's syndrome)
4. EEG (complex partial seizures)
5. Psychometric testing (dementia, schizophrenia, manic-depressive state)
6. Psychiatric consultation

DEPRESSION

Depression may be normal if it is in response to bereavement. It becomes abnormal when it is exaggerated, persistent, or out of proportion to the environment that initiated it. It is usually psychogenic but may be organic.

In the history, is there:
1. **Evidence that the depression is episodic?** Suspect psychomotor epilepsy.
2. **Drug or alcohol abuse?** Chronic use of sedatives, tranquilizers, or narcotics may lead to depression. Alcohol may relieve depression only to lead to worse symptoms on withdrawal.
3. **Insomnia, loss of appetite, impotence, or indecisive behavior?** Consider psychotic depression.
4. **Evidence of menopause?** Consider involutional melancholia.
5. **Occurrence in other members of the family?** Consider manic-depressive psychosis.

On physical examination, is (are) there:
1. **Papilledema or focal neurologic signs?** Consider space-occupying lesion of the brain or multiple sclerosis.
2. **Enlarged thyroid, exophthalmos, tremor, or tachycardia?** Consider apathetic hyperthyroidism.
3. **Hirsutism, centripetal obesity, or purple striae?** Consider Cushing's syndrome.
4. **Evidence of cognitive dysfunction?** Consider senile or presenile dementia.
5. **Tremor and/or rigidity?** Consider Parkinson's disease.

Diagnostic Workup
1. Urine drug screen (drug intoxication)
2. Blood alcohol level (alcoholism)
3. Dexamethasone suppression test (Cushing's syndrome)
4. Free thyroxine and radioiodine uptake and scan (hyperthyroidism)
5. MRI (space-occupying lesion)
6. EEG (psychomotor epilepsy)
7. Serum follicle-stimulating hormone and estradiol (menopause)
8. Psychiatric consultation

DIFFICULTY URINATING

Difficulty may occur in the initiation of urine flow, or the urine stream may be weak or interrupted. The lesion is usually in the lower motor neuron. Difficulty in urination may also be a result of bladder neck obstruction.

In the history, is there:
1. **Pain on voiding?** This would suggest urethritis, cystitis, urethral calculus, urethral carbuncle, or acute prostatitis.
2. **A urethral discharge?** This would indicate acute urethritis or prostatitis.
3. **Weakness or paresthesias in the lower extremities?** Consider spinal cord or cauda equina tumor, herniated disc, multiple sclerosis, tabes dorsalis, spinal cord trauma, or diabetic neuropathy.

On physical examination, is (are) there:
1. **Bladder distention?** This would indicate bladder neck obstruction from prostatic enlargement or urethral stricture.
2. **Enlarged prostate?** This would suggest benign prostatic hypertrophy or advanced prostatic carcinoma. If the prostate is small or firm, consider chronic prostatitis.
3. **Hyperactive or pathologic reflexes in the lower extremities?** Consider multiple sclerosis or spinal cord compression by a space-occupying lesion.
4. **Hypoactive reflexes or atrophy in the lower extremities?** Consider cauda equina tumor, poliomyelitis, radiculopathy, or neuropathy.
5. **Sensory loss?** Consider lesion of the spinal cord, spinal roots, or peripheral nerves.
6. **Tight anal sphincter?** Consider multiple sclerosis or other lesions of the spinal cord.
7. **Weak or relaxed anal sphincter?** Consider cauda equina tumor.

Diagnostic Workup
1. Smear and culture of urethral discharge (gonorrhea, urethritis)
2. Catheterization or ultrasonography for residual urine (urinary retention)
3. Intravenous pyelography (obstructive uropathy)
4. Cystoscopy (urethral stricture, bladder neck obstruction)
5. Cystometric testing (neurogenic bladder)
6. Prostate-specific antigen test (prostatic carcinoma)
7. Venereal Disease Research Laboratory (VDRL) test (syphilis)
8. MRI of the spine (space-occupying lesion of the spinal cord or cauda equina, multiple sclerosis)
9. Neurologic consultation

DIPLOPIA

Diplopia is double vision. The lesion is usually in the brainstem or oculomotor, abducens, or trochlear nerve but may occur in the myoneural junctions or muscles.

In the history, is (are) there:
1. **Involvement of only one eye?** This is a rare occurrence that may be associated with Marfan's disease, congenital double pupil, cataracts, or corneal opacities.
2. **Intermittent symptoms?** Consider myasthenia gravis.
3. **Headache?** Consider space-occupying lesion of the brain or cerebral aneurysm.
4. **Fever?** Consider orbital abscess, brain abscess, cavernous sinus thrombosis, or rarely diphtheria.
5. **Diabetes?** Consider diabetic neuropathy.
6. **Food poisoning?** Consider botulism.

On physical examination, is (are) there:
1. **Proptosis?** Gradual onset of proptosis suggests hyperthyroidism or pituitary exophthalmos. If onset was sudden, consider cavernous sinus thrombosis.
2. **Periorbital edema, chemosis, or ecchymosis?** Consider cavernous sinus thrombosis, orbital tumor or abscess, or arteriovenous aneurysm.
3. **Focal neurologic signs in other cranial nerves or the extremities?** Consider multiple sclerosis, brainstem infarction, or tumor.

Diagnostic Workup
1. Ophthalmologic consultation
2. Neurologic consultation
3. Complete blood count and sedimentation rate (cavernous sinus thrombosis)
4. Radiography of the sinuses and orbits (sinusitis, orbital cellulites)
5. Free thyroxine (hyperthyroidism)
6. Glucose tolerance test (diabetic neuropathy)
7. MRI (brain tumor, multiple sclerosis)
8. Acetylcholine receptor antibody titer (myasthenia gravis)

DIZZINESS

In the history, is there:
1. **True vertigo?** With true vertigo, the patient feels that either he/she or the room is turning, or the patient experiences movement of some kind, especially with the eyes closed and when seated or lying down. If the patient has true vertigo, consider an otologic or a neurologic disorder. If the patient does not have true vertigo, consider a cardiovascular, hematologic, or psychiatric disorder (see Syncope, page 42).
2. **Drug or alcohol use?** Many drugs, including gentamicin, quinine, salicylates, and antihistamines, may cause dizziness or vertigo.
3. **Trauma?** Consider postconcussion syndrome or subdural hematoma.
4. **A recent respiratory or ear infection?** Consider otitis media or acute labyrinthitis (vestibular neuronitis).
5. **Anxiety or depression?** Consider hyperventilation syndrome or other psychiatric disorder.
6. **Tinnitus or deafness?** Consider otitis media, acoustic neuroma, or Meniere's disease.

On physical examination, is (are) there:
1. **Abnormalities on otoscopic examination?** Consider otitis media, impacted cerumen, mastoiditis, petrositis, or cholesteatoma.
2. **Abnormal neurologic findings?** Consider acoustic neuroma or other space-occupying lesion, multiple sclerosis, basilar artery insufficiency or aneurysm, syringobulbia, or platybasia.
3. **Blood pressure abnormalities?** Consider malignant hypertension, postural hypotension, anemia, or cardiovascular disease.
4. **Abnormal cardiac findings?** Consider aortic stenosis, aortic insufficiency, mitral valve disease, congestive heart failure, or cardiac arrhythmia.
5. **Positive Hallpike maneuver?** Consider benign positional vertigo. The Hallpike maneuver is performed by the clinician turning the patient's head to the right while the patient is seated upright. The clinician then abruptly places the patient in the recumbent position with the patient's head over the edge of the examining table while the clinician observes for nystagmus. The procedure is repeated with the patient's head turned to the left.
6. **Pallor?** Consider anemia.

Diagnostic Workup
1. Audiogram and caloric test (acoustic neuroma, Meniere's disease)
2. Neurologic consultation
3. MRI (acoustic neuroma, multiple sclerosis, other brain stem lesions)
4. Spinal tap (neurosyphilis, multiple sclerosis)
5. Brainstem auditory evoked potentials (multiple sclerosis)
6. Magnetic resonance angiography (basilar artery insufficiency)
7. Four-vessel cerebral angiography (cerebrovascular disease)
8. EEG (temporal lobe epilepsy)

EXTREMITY PAIN, LOWER

Lower extremity pain may be focal or diffuse. The lesion is usually in the peripheral nerve, nerve roots, or spinal cord. It also may occur in the joints, bone, or soft tissue.

In the history, is there:
1. **Trauma?** Consider fracture, contusion, or sprain of the lower extremities. Also consider trauma to the joints of the lower extremities. A fracture or herniated disc of the thoracic or lumbar spine may compress the nerve roots causing lower extremity pain.
2. **Unilateral involvement?** This would suggest thrombophlebitis, peripheral artery embolism or thrombosis, fracture, sprain, contusion, cellulitis, or osteomyelitis.
3. **Bilateral involvement?** This would suggest Leriche syndrome, spinal cord or cauda equina lesion, or neurogenic claudication of spinal stenosis.
4. **Sudden onset?** Consider thrombophlebitis, arterial embolism, or cellulitis. If trauma is also involved, consider fracture, sprain, contusion, or torn ligament or meniscus.
5. **Fever?** Consider cellulitis, osteomyelitis, lymphangitis, rheumatic fever, or other infectious disease.

On physical examination, is (are) there:
1. **A focal mass?** Consider cellulitis, abscess, hematoma, or invasive tumor.
2. **Swelling of the involved extremity?** Consider phlebitis or cellulitis.
3. **A positive Homan sign?** Consider deep vein thrombophlebitis.
4. **Diminished or absent pulses?** Consider arterial embolism or thrombosis.
5. **A positive straight leg–raising test or femoral stretch test?** These findings point to a herniated disc of the lumbar spine.
6. **Weakness or sensory deficits?** These suggest myelopathy, radiculopathy, or neuropathy.
7. **Limitation of joint mobility?** Consider hip or knee joint pathology.
8. **Incontinence of urine?** Consider a spinal cord lesion.
9. **Urinary retention?** Consider a cauda equina lesion.

Diagnostic Workup
1. Complete blood count and sedimentation rate (cellulitis, abscess, septic arthritis)
2. Chemistry panel (gout, metastatic cancer).
3. Prostate-specific antigen test (prostatic carcinoma)
4. Synovial fluid analysis (gout, rheumatoid arthritis)
5. Antinuclear antibody analysis (lupus erythematosus)
6. Rheumatoid arthritis titer (rheumatoid arthritis)
7. Radiography of the joints (arthritis)
8. MRI of the joints (torn meniscus)
9. MRI of the spine (herniated disc, neoplasm)
10. Impedance plethysmography or contrast venography (thrombosis)
11. Doppler ultrasonography (thrombophlebitis)
12. Femoral angiography (arterial embolism or thrombosis)
13. Bone scan (osteomyelitis, tumor)
14. Nerve conduction velocity test and electromyography (neuropathy or radiculopathy)

EXTREMITY PAIN, UPPER

Upper extremity pain may be diffuse or focal. The lesion may be in the peripheral nerves, nerve roots, or spinal cord. It may also occur in the sympathetic nerves, joints, or soft tissues.

In the history, is there:

1. **Focal or diffuse pain?** Focal pain may be in or around the joints, in which case the various forms of bursitis, arthritis, and joint trauma must be considered. Focal pain may occur in the bone as a result of fracture, tumor, or osteomyelitis, or it may be a result of cellulitis or contusions. Diffuse pain suggests polymyalgia rheumatica, dermatomyositis, thrombophlebitis, radiculopathy, neuropathy, or sympathetic dystrophy. Rarely, there may be an arterial embolism or thrombosis causing the pain. Referred pain from a myocardial infarct or dissecting aneurysm must be considered.
2. **Trauma?** Consider fracture, contusion, sprain, or torn ligaments. Consider also herniated cervical disc or fracture of the cervical spine.
3. **Fever?** Consider cellulitis, osteomyelitis, rheumatic fever, polymyositis, or systemic infection.
4. **Diabetes mellitus?** Consider peripheral neuropathy.
5. **Tobacco use?** This suggests a Pancoast tumor.
6. **Pain in the face also?** Consider thalamic syndrome.

On physical examination, is (are) there:

1. **Limitation of motion of the shoulder joints?** Consider bursitis, one of the various forms of arthritis, or fractured or torn rotator cuff. Consider also reflex sympathetic dystrophy.
2. **Weakness or paresthesias?** Consider radiculopathy due to a herniated cervical disc or spinal cord lesion. Consider polyneuropathy or mononeuropathy due to carpal tunnel syndrome or ulnar entrapment. Also consider brachial plexus neuritis.
3. **A positive Tinel sign?** A positive Tinel sign at the wrist suggests carpal tunnel syndrome, whereas a positive Tinel sign at the elbow suggests ulnar entrapment.
4. **Neurologic signs in the lower extremities?** Hypoactive reflexes and sensory changes in the lower extremities suggest a peripheral neuropathy, whereas hyperactive reflexes in the lower extremities suggest multiple sclerosis, a cervical cord tumor, or cervical spondylosis.
5. **Positive Adson test?** This suggests a thoracic outlet syndrome.
6. **Vasomotor or tropic changes?** These suggest Raynaud's phenomena or reflex sympathetic dystrophy. Also consider peripheral neuropathy or other collagen diseases.
7. **Swelling?** Consider phlebitis, cellulitis, or lymphatic obstruction.
8. **Absent pulses?** Consider arterial embolism or thrombosis, or dissecting aneurysm.

Diagnostic Workup

1. Complete blood count and sedimentation rate (cellulitis, osteomyelitis, polymyalgia rheumatica)
2. Antinuclear antibody test (collagen disease)
3. Rheumatoid arthritis titer (rheumatoid arthritis)
4. Chemistry panel (gout)
5. Radiography of the joints (fracture, arthritis)
6. Radiography of the cervical spine (fracture, herniated disc)
7. MRI of the shoulder (torn rotator cuff)
8. MRI of the cervical spine (herniated disc, tumor)
9. Bone scan (osteomyelitis, invasive tumor)
10. Nerve conduction velocity test and electromyography (neuropathy, radiculopathy, polymyositis)
11. Exercise tolerance test (coronary insufficiency)
12. Stellate ganglion block (reflex sympathetic dystrophy)
13. Venography (thrombophlebitis)
14. Arteriography (arterial occlusion)
15. Neurologic consultation
16. Orthopedic consultation

EYE PAIN

The definition of eye pain is self-evident. The location of the lesion is most likely in the eye, sinuses, optic nerve, trigeminal nerve, brain, or arteries.

In the history, is there:
1. **Trauma?** Consider concussion, skull fracture of the floor of the orbit or maxillary sinus, corneal abrasion, or retinal detachment.
2. **A discharge?** Consider conjunctivitis, foreign body, or refractive error.
3. **Headache?** Eye pain is frequently associated with migraine or cluster headache.
4. **Sinusitis?** Sinusitis is a frequent cause of eye pain.
5. **Fever?** Local and systemic infections cause eye pain.

On physical examination, is (are) there:
1. **Redness of the eye?** Consider conjunctivitis, keratitis, foreign body, iritis, or glaucoma.
2. **Visual field defect without visible changes of the eyeball?** Consider optic neuritis.
3. **Periorbital edema?** Consider orbital cellulitis, neoplasm, cavernous sinus thrombosis, or arteriovenous aneurysm.
4. **Rash of the eyelid?** Consider herpes zoster ophthalmicus.
5. **Increased intraocular pressure?** Consider glaucoma.
6. **A refractive error?** Myopia and astigmatism are a frequent cause of eye pain, especially in the evening.
7. **Papilledema?** Consider optic neuritis, hypertension, or a space-occupying lesion of the brain.
8. **Proptosis?** Consider Grave's disease, orbital tumor, arteriovenous aneurysm, or cavernous sinus thrombosis.
9. **Other neurologic signs?** Consider multiple sclerosis, brain tumor, or stroke.

Diagnostic Workup
1. Smear and culture of exudate (conjunctivitis, cellulitis)
2. Fluorescein dye test (foreign body, abrasion)
3. Tonometry (glaucoma)
4. Slit lamp examination (iritis, keratitis)
5. Visual field examination (optic neuritis, glaucoma)
6. Radiography of sinuses (sinusitis)
7. Ophthalmologic consultation
8. Neurologic consultation
9. MRI or CT scan (brain tumor)

FACIAL PAIN

The definition of facial pain is self-evident. The location of the lesion is most likely in the face, trigeminal nerve, or brainstem, but the lesion may also occur in the arteries.

In the history, is there:
1. **Trauma?** Consider fracture or contusion of the sinuses, orbit, or mandible.
2. **Stabbing, shooting pain?** Consider trigeminal neuralgia, typical migraine, multiple sclerosis, or thalamic syndrome.
3. **Throbbing pain?** Consider migraine or cluster headache.
4. **Constant pain of gradual onset?** Consider tumor or other space-occupying lesion of the posterior fossa.
5. **Fever?** Consider acute sinusitis or dental abscess.
6. **Nasal discharge?** Consider sinus abscess or cluster headache.
7. **An elderly patient?** Consider trigeminal neuralgia.
8. **Precipitation of the pain by chewing?** Consider temporomandibular joint syndrome or trigeminal neuralgia.
9. **Pain that occurs at night?** Consider cluster headache.

On physical examination, is (are) there:
1. **A rash?** Consider herpes zoster.
2. **A swollen, tender temporal artery?** Consider temporal arteritis.
3. **A swollen, tender temporomandibular joint with dental malocclusion?** Consider temporomandibular joint syndrome.
4. **Poor transillumination of the sinuses?** Consider acute sinusitis.
5. **Relief of the pain with sumatriptan?** Consider migraine or cluster headache.
6. **Abnormal neurologic findings?** Consider posterior fossa tumor, multiple sclerosis, or Wallenberg syndrome.

Diagnostic Workup
1. Complete blood count (sinusitis)
2. Sedimentation rate (temporal arteritis)
3. Radiography of the sinuses (acute sinusitis)
4. Radiography of the temporomandibular joints or SPECT scan (temporomandibular joint syndrome)
5. Radiography of the teeth (dental abscess)
6. MRI or CT scan (space-occupying lesion, multiple sclerosis)
7. Angiography (Wallenberg syndrome)
8. Histamine test (cluster headache)
9. Response to sumatriptan (migraine, cluster headache)
10. Trial of anticonvulsants (trigeminal neuralgia)
11. Ear, nose, and throat consultation (sinusitis)
12. Neurologic consultation
13. Dental consultation

Treatment
Trigeminal neuralgia is treated first with anticonvulsants, as more than half the patients respond to carbamazepine (Tegretol; Novartis, East Hanover, NJ); see Appendix C for dosages. If there is no response to anticonvulsant medication, alcohol or boiling water may be injected into the maxillary or mandibular branches of the trigeminal nerve. Because there is more than one surgical procedure available for definitive treatment of this disorder, a neurosurgeon should be consulted.

HALLUCINATIONS

Hallucinations are sensations, usually auditory or visual, that are spontaneous and not based on any external stimulation. The lesion is psychogenic, or it may occur in the cerebrum.

In the history, is (are) there:
1. **Evidence of drug use or abuse?** Many illegal drugs may produce hallucinations, including cocaine, amphetamines, marijuana, lysergic acid diethylamide (LSD), and heroin. Prescription drugs associated with hallucinations include the tricyclic antidepressants, anti-Parkinson drugs such as levodopa, and narcotics.
2. **A seizure disorder?** Temporal lobe epilepsy may be associated with hallucinations or déjà vu phenomena.
3. **Depression?** Psychotic depressive states may be associated with hallucinations.
4. **Alcohol consumption?** Both acute and chronic alcohol consumption may produce hallucinations. Withdrawal from alcohol produces the well-known delirium tremens and visual and auditory hallucinations.
5. **Flattened or disturbed affect, ambivalence, or autism?** Consider schizophrenia.
6. **Episodic hallucinations with normal periods in between?** Consider primary epilepsy or symptomatic epilepsy due to a space-occupying lesion.
7. **Episodes of falling asleep during the day?** This would suggest the hypnagogic hallucinations of narcolepsy.

On physical examination, is (are) there:
1. **Focal neurologic signs?** Consider a space-occupying lesion such as brain tumor or hematoma.
2. **Mental deterioration?** Consider Alzheimer's disease or cerebral arteriosclerosis.

Diagnostic Workup
1. Blood alcohol level (alcohol intoxication)
2. Urine drug screen (drug intoxication)
3. Psychiatric consultation (schizophrenia)
4. MRI (space-occupying lesion)
5. EEG, awake and asleep (epilepsy)
6. Psychometric testing (dementia)
7. Sleep study (narcolepsy)

HEADACHE

In the history is (are) there:

1. **Acute onset?** This should prompt consideration of migraine, subarachnoid hemorrhage, meningitis, temporal arteritis, cluster headaches, or infectious disease.
2. **Chronic onset?** Consider tension headache, post-traumatic headache, hypertension, or space-occupying lesion.
3. **Focal headache?** Consider migraine, temporal arteritis, glaucoma, space-occupying lesion, or cluster headache.
4. **Diffuse headache?** Consider tension headache, common migraine, post-traumatic headache, meningitis, subarachnoid hemorrhage, or pseudotumor cerebri.
5. **Throbbing headache?** Consider migraine, hypertensive headache, temporal arteritis, arteriovenous anomaly.
6. **Nausea and vomiting?** Consider migraine, brain tumor, malignant hypertension, meningitis, or subarachnoid hemorrhage.
7. **Fever?** Consider meningitis or other infectious disease, temporal arteritis, or cerebral hemorrhage.
8. **Drug, caffeine, or alcohol use?** Consider drug-induced or withdrawal headache, or subdural hematoma (due to secondary trauma).

On physical examination, is (are) there:

1. **Papilledema?** Consider space-occupying lesion (e.g., tumor), malignant hypertension, or pseudotumor cerebri.
2. **Focal neurologic signs?** Consider space-occupying lesion or stroke.
3. **Nuchal rigidity?** Consider meningitis or subarachnoid hemorrhage.
4. **Tender or enlarged temporal artery?** Consider temporal arteritis.
5. **Increased intraocular tension?** Consider glaucoma.
6. **Poor transillumination of the sinuses?** Consider acute or chronic sinusitis.
7. **Poor range of motion of the neck?** Consider cervical spondylosis, meningitis, or subarachnoid hemorrhage.
8. **Hypertension?** Consider hypertensive headache or pheochromocytoma.
9. **Infection elsewhere?** Consider brain abscess or meningitis.

Diagnostic Workup

1. Complete blood count (infectious disease)
2. Chemistry panel (toxic encephalopathy)
3. Drug screen (drug intoxication)
4. Blood alcohol level (alcoholism)
5. Venereal Disease Research Laboratory (VDRL) test (neurosyphilis)
6. Sedimentation rate (temporal arteritis)
7. Radiography of the sinuses (sinusitis)
8. Radiography of cervical spine (cervical spondylosis)
9. CT scan (space-occupying lesion, subarachnoid hemorrhage
10. MRI (space-occupying lesion)
11. Spinal tap (meninigitis, subarachnoid hemorrhage)
12. Cerebral angiography (aneurysm, arteriovenous anomaly)
13. Therapeutic trial (migraine, see Appendix C)
14. Neurologic consultation

HEAD MASS OR SWELLING

A head mass or swelling may be focal or diffuse. The lesion may be localized to the skin, subcutaneous tissue, skull, meninges, or brain.

In the history, is there:
1. **Trauma?** Consider extracranial or intracranial hematoma.
2. **Evidence of a difficult delivery?** Consider a cephalhematoma or edema of the scalp (caput succedaneum).

On physical examination, is there:
1. **A focal mass?** Consider sebaceous cyst, lipoma, lymph node, hematoma, osteoma, meningocele, or malignant tumor.
2. **A diffuse mass?** Consider hematoma, edema, hydrocephalus, meningocele, tumor, or vascular abnormality.
3. **Fixation to the skull?** Consider Paget's disease, osteoma, sarcoma, multiple myeloma, subperiosteal hematoma, or enlarged sutures. Meningoceles are also fixed.
4. **A freely movable mass?** Consider sebaceous cyst or lymph node, lipoma, or small hematoma or abscess.

Diagnostic Workup
1. Radiography of the skull (osteoma, multiple myeloma, metastasis, meningioma)
2. CT scan (space-occupying lesion of the brain or skull)
3. Neurologic consultation
4. Surgical consultation

HIP PAIN

The lesion is usually in the hip, around the hip, or in the peripheral nerve or nerve roots.

In the history, is there:
1. **Trauma?** Consider fracture, contusion, or sprain or strain of the hip joint. Also consider a herniated lumbar disc or vertebral fracture with compression of the sciatic nerve roots.
2. **Fever?** Consider subcutaneous abscess osteomyelitis, rheumatic fever, or septic arthritis.
3. **Involvement of other joints?** Consider gout, rheumatoid arthritis, osteoarthritis, or rheumatic fever.
4. **A young age?** Consider congenital dislocation of the joint, slipped femoral epiphysis, or Legg-Calvé-Perthes disease.
5. **Use of corticosteroids?** Consider vascular necrosis.

On physical examination, is (are) there:
1. **A tender greater trochanter bursa?** Consider greater trochanter bursitis.
2. **A mass?** Consider abscess, hematoma, tumor, osteomyelitis, or fracture/dislocation.
3. **Limitation of motion of the joint?** This would indicate a hip fracture, osteoarthritis, rheumatoid arthritis, gout or sepsis of the joint, a slipped femoral epiphysis, or Legg-Calvé-Perthes disease.
4. **A rash?** Consider herpes zoster.
5. **A positive Patrick test?** This would suggest arthritis of the hip or greater trochanter bursitis. It could also suggest other types of hip pathology mentioned above.
6. **A positive straight leg–raising test?** Consider a herniated lumbar disc with radiculopathy.
7. **Hypoactive reflexes or motor or sensory finding of the involved lower extremity?** This would suggest a herniated disc, vertebral fracture, or cauda equina tumor.

Diagnostic Workup
1. Complete blood count (septic arthritis)
2. Sedimentation rate (infection, rheumatic fever, rheumatoid arthritis)
3. Chemistry panel (gout, pseudogout)
4. Rheumatoid arthritis test (rheumatoid arthritis)
5. Radiography of the hip (fracture, dislocation, arthritis)
6. Radiography of the lumbar spine (fracture, herniated disc)
7. Bone scan (osteomyelitis, tumor)
8. CT scan or MRI of the hip (fracture, neoplasm)
9. MRI of the lumbar spine (herniated disc, neoplasm)
10. Lidocaine injection to the greater trochanter bursa (greater trochanter bursitis)
11. Orthopedic consultation
12. Neurologic consultation

HOARSENESS

Hoarseness varies from a distortion to a complete absence of the voice. The lesion is most often in the vocal cords, peripheral nerve, or brainstem. It may be psychogenic.

In the history, is there:
1. **A gradual or acute onset?** A gradual onset of hoarseness would suggest a neoplasm of the larynx or mediastinal mass such as a tumor or aneurysm compressing the recurrent laryngeal nerve. Hypothyroidism also may cause a gradual onset of hoarseness. An acute onset would suggest trauma, infection, or allergy as the etiology.
2. **Intermittent occurrence of the hoarseness?** This suggests vocal abuse from various occupations or myasthenia gravis. Alcohol and tobacco abuse may produce intermittent hoarseness.
3. **Associated chronic cough or hemoptysis?** Consider bronchogenic carcinoma, carcinoma of the larynx, tuberculosis, or fungal infection.
4. **A chronic nasal or postnasal drip?** Consider chronic sinusitis.
5. **Chronic heartburn?** Consider reflux esophagitis.

On physical examination is (are) there:
1. **A mass or ulceration of the vocal cords?** Consider carcinoma, singer's nodes, tuberculosis, or syphilis.
2. **Vocal cord paralysis?** Consider carcinoma of the lung, aortic aneurysm, mediastinal tumor, thyroid tumor, or brainstem lesion.
3. **Abnormal neurologic signs in the cranial nerve or extremities?** Consider stroke, Guillain-Barré syndrome, or brainstem tumor.
4. **Relief on administration of edrophonium (Tensilon; ICN Pharmaceuticals, Costa Mesa, CA)?** Consider myasthenia gravis.

Diagnostic Workup
1. Complete blood count and sedimentation test (laryngitis)
2. Venereal Disease Research Laboratory (VDRL) test (syphilis)
3. Tuberculin test (tuberculosis)
4. Radiography of the chest (pneumonia, tuberculosis, neoplasm)
5. Thyroid function tests (myxedema)
6. CT scan of the chest (tumor of the lung or mediastinum)
7. CT scan or MRI of the brain (brainstem tumor)
8. Aortography (aortic aneurysm)
9. Radioiodine uptake and scan (thyroid tumor)
10. Allergy skin test (allergy).

HYPERSOMNIA

Hypersomnia is the desire for and act of sleeping more than necessary. The lesion is in the brain or brainstem; it may also be psychogenic.

In the history, is (are) there:
1. **Loss of appetite or libido, or depression?** These symptoms are typical of endogenous depression.
2. **Hallucinations, cataplexy, or sleep paralysis?** These symptoms are typical of narcolepsy. The hallucinations are auditory or visual and occur halfway between waking and sleep (so-called hypnagogic), especially at night. Cataplexy is a sudden loss of muscle tone associated with laughter or surprise. Sleep paralysis is the sudden inability to move the extremities upon awakening from sleep. Narcolepsy may be symptomatic of a postconcussion syndrome, a brain tumor, multiple sclerosis, or trypanosomiasis.
3. **Diabetes or uremia?** Hypersomnia may herald the onset of diabetic or uremic coma.
4. **Associated hunger or restlessness with the attacks?** This may indicate the rare Kleine-Levin syndrome in young adults.
5. **Drug or alcohol use?** Chronic abuse of barbiturates or alcohol may cause hypersomnia.

On physical examination, are there:
1. **Focal neurologic signs?** Consider multiple sclerosis, neurosyphilis, or space-occupying lesion of the brain.

Diagnostic Workup
1. Complete blood count and sedimentation rate (encephalitis)
2. Venereal Disease Research Laboratory (VDRL) test (neurosyphilis)
3. Chemistry panel (diabetes mellitus, uremia)
4. Urine drug screen (drug intoxication, alcoholism)
5. Sleep study (narcolepsy, epilepsy)
6. MRI (brain tumor, multiple sclerosis)
7. Spinal tap (multiple sclerosis, neurosyphilis, encephalitis)
8. Neurologic consultation
9. Psychiatric consultation

IMPOTENCE

Impotence is the inability to obtain or maintain an erection, whereas sterility is the inability to have children. The lesion causing impotence may be in the brain, spinal cord, peripheral nerves, or end organ.

In the history, is (are) there:

1. **Pressure on the job, at school, or in the personal relationship, especially from a dissatisfied or dominating partner?** This may cause physiologic or psychological impotence.
2. **Alcohol abuse?** Alcohol promotes sexual desire but may prevent completion of the act.
3. **Drug use or abuse?** Many prescription drugs may induce partial or complete impotence. These include antihypertensive drugs such as beta-blockers, methyldopa, and guanethidine, as well as the tricyclic antidepressants and benzodiazepines such as diazepine. Almost any prescription drug with sedative effects may cause impotence. Impotence is also caused by nicotine and narcotics and other illegal drugs.
4. **Diabetes?** Diabetic neuropathy is a frequent cause of impotence.
5. **Anxiety or depression?** Most cases of impotence are a result of a psychological disorder.
6. **Weakness or paresthesias in the extremities?** Impotence is associated with many neurologic disorders, most notably, peripheral neuropathy, multiple sclerosis, spinal cord injury and tumors, and tabes dorsalis.
7. **Incontinence or difficulty voiding?** This may signify a urologic or neurologic disorder.

On physical examination, is (are) there:

1. **Loss of secondary sex characteristics?** Consider Fröhlich's syndrome, Klinefelter's syndrome, or other congenital disorder.
2. **Enlarged or firm prostate?** Chronic prostatitis, prostatic hypertrophy, and prostatic carcinoma may cause impotence.
3. **Small testes?** Testicular atrophy may be associated with impotence.
4. **Other genital abnormalities?** Peyronie's disease may cause painful erections and thus lead to impotence.
5. **Hyperactive or pathologic reflexes?** Look for multiple sclerosis or a spinal cord or brainstem disorder.
6. **Hypoactive reflexes and sensory loss?** Look for peripheral neuropathy, tabes dorsalis, or pernicious anemia.
7. **Poor pulses in the lower extremities?** Consider Leriche syndrome or peripheral arteriosclerosis.

Diagnostic Workup

1. Urine drug screen (drug intoxication)
2. Urinalysis and urine culture (urinary tract infection)
3. Chemistry panel (diabetes mellitus, uremia)
4. Venereal Disease Research Laboratory (VDRL) test (tabes dorsalis)
5. Thyroid profile (hypothyroidism)
6. Serum testosterone and gonadotropin assay (testicular atrophy, Klinefelter's syndrome)
7. Nerve conduction velocity studies (peripheral neuropathy)
8. Somatosensory evoked potential mapping (multiple sclerosis)
9. MRI of the spine (tumor, multiple sclerosis)
10. Spinal tap (multiple sclerosis, neurosyphilis)
11. Urologic consultation (prostatic carcinoma, bladder neck obstruction)
12. Penile blood pressure studies (arteriosclerosis)
13. Nocturnal tumescent study (diabetic neuropathy)
14. Aortography (Leriche syndrome)

INCONTINENCE OF FECES

Incontinence of feces is the involuntary release of stool in an inappropriate time and/or place. The lesion is usually in the spinal cord or peripheral nerve, but fecal incontinence may also be caused by end-organ disorders or dementia.

In the history, is (are) there:
1. **Rectal surgery?** Hemorrhoidectomy or surgery for a rectal fissure may leave the anal sphincter in a dysfunctional state.
2. **Trauma?** Trauma to the spinal cord may cause bilateral pyramidal tract damage leading to incontinence of feces.
3. **Drug or alcohol abuse?** Incontinence may result from heavy intoxication with drugs or alcohol.
4. **Infrequent episodes?** Consider epilepsy or organic brain syndrome.

On physical examination, is (are) there:
1. **Hyperactive or pathologic reflexes?** Consider spinal cord tumor, multiple sclerosis, or transverse myelitis.
2. **Hypoactive reflexes?** Consider cauda equina tumor, tabes dorsalis, spinal stenosis, or other disease of the lumbosacral spine.
3. **Local disease of the anus?** Consider anal fissure, anal fistula, hemorrhoids, or carcinoma.

Diagnostic Workup
1. Anoscopy (hemorrhoids, carcinoma)
2. Radiography of the lumbar spine (spinal stenosis, metastatic carcinoma)
3. MRI of the brain or spinal cord (tumor, multiple sclerosis)
4. Spinal fluid examination (multiple sclerosis, neurosyphilis)
5. EEG (epilepsy)
6. Anorectal manometry (rectal muscle dysfunction)

INCONTINENCE OF URINE

Incontinence of urine is the involuntary release of urine at an inappropriate time and/or place. The lesion is usually in the spinal cord or lumbosacral nerve roots but may occur in the end organ or brain.

In the history, is (are) there:
1. **Urologic surgery?** Incontinence of urine may occur after surgery to the bladder neck or prostate.
2. **Trauma?** Trauma to the spinal cord may lead to incontinence.
3. **Drug or alcohol use or abuse?** Heavy drug or alcohol intoxication is associated with incontinence.
4. **Infrequent episodes?** Consider epilepsy or transient ischemic attack.
5. **Incontinence only on coughing or increasing abdominal pressure?** Consider stress incontinence.
6. **Burning on urination, urethral discharge, or hematuria?** These findings would suggest cystitis or urethritis as the cause of the incontinence.

On physical examination, is (are) there:
1. **A distended bladder?** Consider overflow incontinence from a bladder neck obstruction.
2. **Enlarged prostate?** Consider benign prostatic hypertrophy or carcinoma of the prostate.
3. **Hyperactive or pathologic reflexes in the lower extremities?** Consider spinal cord tumor, multiple sclerosis, or transverse myelitis.
4. **Hypoactive reflexes in the lower extremities?** Consider cauda equina tumor, spinal stenosis, or diabetic neuropathy.
5. **Ataxia with dementia?** Consider normal pressure hydrocephalus.
6. **A cystocele or rectocele?** Consider stress incontinence.

Diagnostic Workup
1. Urinalysis and urine culture (cystitis, urinary tract infection)
2. Catheterization for residual urine (bladder neck obstruction)
3. Perineal pad test (stress incontinence)
4. Q-tip test (stress incontinence)
5. Sonography to test for residual urine
6. Cystoscopy (bladder carcinoma, bladder neck obstruction)
7. Cystometric testing to differentiate between spastic and flaccid neurogenic bladder
8. CT scan of lumbar spine (cauda equina tumor)
9. MRI of brain and/or spinal cord (multiple sclerosis, tumor)
10. Nerve conduction velocity test and electromyography (neuropathy)
11. Urologic consultation
12. Neurologic consultation

INSOMNIA

Insomnia is the inability to fall asleep and maintain sleep for a normal period of time, usually considered to be 6 to 8 hours. However, what is considered normal may vary among individuals with respect to age and other factors. The lesion occurs in the cerebrum or is supratentorial, but insomnia may be caused by severe pain from any disorder or from respiratory distress or cardiopulmonary disorders.

In the history, is there:

1. **Loss of appetite or libido?** Depression is a common cause of insomnia. Chronic anxiety often prevents sleep.
2. **Drug or alcohol abuse?** Narcotics, amphetamines, and alcohol may cause insomnia, especially during the withdrawal phase. Obviously, caffeine is a prominent cause, and elderly patients are particularly vulnerable.
3. **Shortness of breath?** Congestive heart failure and chronic respiratory disorders cause insomnia.
4. **Chronic pain?** Arthritis, dental abscess, a herniated disc, reflux esophagitis, and angina pectoris are just a few of the painful conditions that disturb sleep.

On physical examination, is (are) there:

1. **A rash?** Eczema, contact dermatitis, dermatophytosis, exfoliative dermatitis, and dermatitis herpetiformis are just a few of the skin conditions that may cause insomnia.
2. **Dementia?** Alzheimer's disease and cerebral arteriosclerosis are associated with insomnia.
3. **Sibilant or sonorous rales?** Look for asthma or emphysema.
4. **Crepitant rales?** These suggest congestive heart failure.
5. **Elevated blood pressure?** Hypertension may be associated with insomnia.

Diagnostic Workup

1. Complete blood count (anemia)
2. Chemistry panel (diabetes, uremia)
3. Pulmonary function tests (emphysema, congestive heart failure)
4. Urine drug screen (drug intoxication)
5. Thyroid profile (hyperthyroidism)
6. 24-hour urine catecholamines (pheochromocytoma)
7. Polysomnography (sleep apnea)
8. MRI of the brain (Alzheimer's disease)
9. Psychiatric consultation

MEMORY LOSS

The definition of memory loss is self-evident, but loss of memory of recent events or poor memory retention is what causes the patient or family member to seek medical help. The lesion is located in the supratentorial region of the brain.

In the history, is there:
1. **Trauma?** Consider concussion or subdural hematoma. These conditions need to be considered even if there is no history of trauma.
2. **Drug or alcohol use or abuse?** Although many prescription drugs may impair memory, illegal drugs such as lysergic acid diethylamide (LSD) and phencyclidine (PCP) cause the most serious memory loss. Chronic alcoholism may produce Korsakoff syndrome or Wernicke's encephalopathy.
3. **Depression or anxiety?** Patients with depressive disorders or chronic anxiety often complain of memory loss, but this observation is more subjective than objective in nature. Dissociative reaction is a neurosis that is associated with memory loss.
4. **Menopause?** Involutional melancholia is associated with subjective memory loss.
5. **Secondary gain?** Look for malingering.
6. **High-risk sexual behavior?** Consider acquired immunodeficiency syndrome encephalitis.

On physical examination, is (are) there:
1. **Pallor?** Pernicious anemia may be associated with memory loss.
2. **Nonpitting edema?** Hypothyroidism may cause memory loss.
3. **Tremor or rigidity?** Parkinson syndrome and other extrapyramidal disorders are associated with memory loss. Manganese toxicity may also produce tremor, rigidity, and memory loss.
4. **Papilledema or focal neurologic signs?** Look for brain tumor, multiple sclerosis, cerebral infarction, or other space-occupying lesion.
5. **Unusual odor to breath?** Look for hepatic or uremic encephalopathy.
6. **Pathologic mouth-opening response or grasp and after-grasp reflexes?** Consider Alzheimer's disease.

Diagnostic Workup
1. Complete blood count and serum vitamin B_{12} analysis (pernicious anemia)
2. Sedimentation rate (viral encephalitis)
3. Venereal Disease Research Laboratory (VDRL) test (neurosyphilis)
4. Chemistry panel (uremia, hepatic failure)
5. Thyroid profile (myxedema)
6. Urine drug screen (drug intoxication)
7. Blood alcohol level (chronic alcoholism)
8. MRI (brain tumor, multiple sclerosis, Alzheimer's disease)
9. EEG (seizure disorders, drug intoxication)
10. Cerebral angiography (cerebral infarct)
11. Spinal tap (neurosyphilis, multiple sclerosis)
12. Psychiatric consultation
13. Human immunodeficiency virus antibody (acquired immunodeficiency syndrome).

NECK PAIN

Neck pain may be defined as pain anywhere between the base of the head and shoulders. The lesion is usually located in the spinal cord, meninges, nerve roots, or brachial plexus. The pain may be referred from the heart or great vessels.

In the history, is there:
1. **Trauma?** Consider cervical sprain, herniated disc, vertebral fracture, or spinal cord trauma.
2. **Fever?** Consider meningitis and subarachnoid hemorrhage. Also consider systemic infections and subdiaphragmatic abscess.
3. **Headache?** Cervical pain may be secondary to migraine, muscle contraction headache, or a space-occupying lesion of the brain.
4. **Heart disease?** Consider coronary insufficiency.
5. **Joint pain or stiffness in the extremities?** Consider rheumatoid arthritis or osteoarthritis.
6. **Radiation of pain into the upper extremities?** Consider radiculopathy due to herniated disc, cervical spondylosis, or spinal cord tumor.

On physical examination, is (are) there:
1. **A mass?** Consider a Pancoast tumor, abscess, Hodgkin's disease, aneurysm, thyroid tumor, or acute thyroiditis.
2. **Nuchal rigidity?** Consider meningitis or subarachnoid hemorrhage.
3. **Hypoactive reflexes or dermatomal sensory loss in the upper extremities?** Consider herniated disc, brachial plexus neuritis, cervical spondylosis, or early spinal cord tumor.
4. **Hyperactive reflexes in the lower extremities?** Consider cervical spondylosis, vertebral fracture, space-occupying lesion of the cervical spinal cord, or midline cervical disc herniation.

Diagnostic Workup
1. Complete blood count and sedimentation rate (abscess)
2. Serum protein electrophoresis (multiple myeloma)
3. Thyroid profile (acute thyroiditis)
4. Arthritis panel (rheumatoid arthritis)
5. Radiography of the cervical spine (cervical spondylosis)
6. Bone scan (metastatic carcinoma, osteomyelitis)
7. MRI (herniated disc, spinal cord tumor)
8. Electromyography and nerve conduction velocity study (brachial plexus neuritis, injury, or herniated disc)
9. Chest radiography (bronchogenic carcinoma, tuberculosis, mediastinal tumor)
10. Neurologic consultation

NIGHTMARES

Nightmares are vivid dreams that terrify the subject and are clearly remembered long after the event. The lesion is in the brain or supratentorial area (psychogenic).

In the history, is there:
1. **Trauma?** Surgery and head trauma may precipitate nightmares.
2. **Fever?** Any systemic infection associated with fever may precipitate nightmares.
3. **Drug or alcohol use or abuse?** Certain prescription drugs, such as benzodiazepines, may cause nightmares. Alcohol withdrawal, particularly delirium tremens, may be associated with nightmares.
4. **Anxiety or pressure on the job, at school, or in the home?** Normal and abnormal fears may provoke nightmares.
5. **Incontinence or tongue biting?** Consider nocturnal attacks of epilepsy.

On physical examination, is (are) there:
1. **Lacerations of the tongue?** Look for epilepsy.
2. **Needle tracks?** Consider drug use.
3. **Rash?** Consider systemic disease.

Diagnostic Workup
1. Complete blood count and sedimentation rate (infectious disease)
2. Urine drug screen (drug intoxication)
3. Blood alcohol level (alcoholism)
4. EEG, awake and asleep (epilepsy)
5. Psychometric testing (chronic anxiety neurosis)
6. Psychiatric consultation

PARESTHESIAS OF THE EXTREMITIES

Paresthesias may be described as numbness, tingling, or distorted sensations in the skin. The lesion may be located in the peripheral nerve, nerve root, spinal cord, brainstem, or brain.

In the history, is (are) there:
1. **Pain in the extremity?** Consider involvement of the nerve root by a herniated disc, spondylosis, fracture of the spine, or space-occupying lesion.
2. **Headache?** Consider space-occupying lesion of the brain or migraine.
3. **Intermittent occurrence?** Consider migraine, epilepsy, or transient ischemic attack.
4. **Trauma?** Consider hematoma or contusion of the brain or spinal cord.
5. **Drug or alcohol use?** Consider toxic or metabolic neuropathy.
6. **Visual disturbances?** Consider multiple sclerosis or migraine.
7. **Incontinence?** Consider multiple sclerosis or spinal cord disorder.
8. **Urinary retention?** Consider cauda equina lesion.

On physical examination, is (are) there:
1. **Papilledema?** Consider space-occupying lesion of the brain or brainstem.
2. **Visual field defect?** Consider space-occupying lesion, cerebrovascular disease, or multiple sclerosis.
3. **Diminished pulses in the involved extremity?** Consider peripheral arteriosclerosis or major artery obstruction.
4. **Hypoactive reflexes in the involved extremity?** Consider herniated disc, neuropathy, or plexopathy.
5. **Hyperactive reflexes in the involved extremities?** Consider multiple sclerosis, pernicious anemia, or spinal cord, brain, or brainstem lesion.
6. **Cranial nerve signs?** Consider multiple sclerosis, cerebrovascular disease, or space-occupying lesion of the brain or brainstem.
7. **Dermatomal sensory loss?** Consider herniated disc or other space-occupying lesion of the nerve root.
8. **Tinel's sign of the wrist?** Consider carpal tunnel syndrome.
9. **Tinel's sign of the elbow?** Consider ulnar entrapment.
10. **Positive straight leg–raising test?** Consider herniated disc of L4-L5 or L5-S1 level.
11. **Positive femoral stretch test?** Consider herniated disc of L3-L4.
12. **Positive Adson's test?** Consider thoracic outlet syndrome.

Diagnostic Workup
1. Complete blood count (pernicious anemia)
2. Chemistry panel (diabetic neuropathy)
3. Venereal Disease Research Laboratory (VDRL) test (neurosyphilis)
4. Plain films of the cervical or lumbar spine (fracture, herniated disc, tumor, etc.)
5. Serum protein electrophoresis (multiple myeloma)
6. Urine porphobilinogen (porphyria)
7. MRI of the spinal cord (herniated disc, tumor, multiple sclerosis)
8. MRI of the brain (space-occupying lesion, cerebrovascular disease, multiple sclerosis)
9. Somatosensory evoked potentials (multiple sclerosis)
10. Nerve conduction velocity studies (peripheral neuropathy, carpal tunnel syndrome, etc.)
11. Spinal tap (multiple sclerosis, neurosyphilis)
12. Heavy metal screen (neuropathy)
13. Serum vitamin B_{12} analysis (pernicious anemia)

PHOTOPHOBIA

Photophobia is sensitivity of the eyes to light. The lesion is usually located in the eye itself, but photophobia may be caused by a systemic disorder.

In the history, is (are) there:
1. **Burning or pain in the eye?** Consider conjunctivitis, keratitis, iritis, glaucoma, or foreign body.
2. **Blurred vision?** Consider refractive error, astigmatism, glaucoma, or uveitis.
3. **Fever?** Consider meningitis or a systemic infection such as measles.
4. **Recurrent headaches?** Photophobia is a common symptom of migraine headaches.
5. **Drug use?** Cocaine and amphetamine use are commonly associated with photophobia, but any drug that dilates the pupils may produce the same effects.

On physical examination, is (are) there:
1. **A red eye?** Consider conjunctivitis, foreign body, keratitis, iritis, scleritis, or glaucoma.
2. **An ocular discharge?** Consider conjunctivitis, corneal ulcer, foreign body, or migraine.
3. **Dilated pupils?** Consider glaucoma or drug use.
4. **Constricted pupils?** Consider iritis.
5. **Nuchal rigidity?** Consider meningitis or subarachnoid hemorrhage.
6. **Lack of pigment in hair, skin, and eyes?** Consider albinism.

Diagnostic Workup
1. Complete blood count and sedimentation rate (systemic infection)
2. Urine drug screen (drug intoxication)
3. Tonometry (glaucoma)
4. Slit lamp examination (iritis, keratitis)
5. Histamine test (migraine, cluster headache)
6. Ophthalmologic consultation
7. Neurologic consultation
8. Trial of beta-blockers (migraine)

RESTLESS LEGS SYNDROME

Restless legs syndrome is the sensation of burning, prickling, tickling, or crawling in the lower extremities, usually occurring at night. It is difficult for individuals with this syndrome to find a comfortable position for their legs. The lesion is usually in the spinal cord, nerve roots, or peripheral nerve but may occur in the extrapyramidal system.

In the history, is there:
1. **Drug or alcohol use?** Consider the use of amphetamines, benzodiazepines, cocaine, caffeine, or various tranquilizers. Withdrawal from alcohol may also produce restless legs syndrome.
2. **Diabetes?** Restless legs syndrome may be associated with diabetic neuropathy.
3. **Back pain?** Consider herniated disc or other disease of the nerve roots.

On physical examination, is (are) there:
1. **Pallor?** Consider anemia.
2. **Hypoactive reflexes or glove and stocking hypalgesia or hypesthesia?** Consider peripheral neuropathy.
3. **Hyperactive reflexes?** Consider multiple sclerosis or other lesion of the spinal cord.
4. **Tremor or rigidity?** Consider Parkinsonian syndrome.
5. **Poor peripheral pulses?** Consider peripheral arteriosclerosis or Leriche syndrome.

Diagnostic Workup
1. Complete blood count (anemia)
2. Serum vitamin B_{12} analysis (pernicious anemia)
3. Chemistry panel (diabetes, uremia)
4. Urine drug screen (drug intoxication)
5. Doppler studies (peripheral arteriosclerosis)
6. Nerve conduction velocity studies (peripheral neuropathy)
7. MRI of the spine (multiple sclerosis)
8. Pregnancy test
9. Neurologic consultation

SCOTOMA

A scotoma is a localized defect in the visual field. It is usually perceived as a blind spot but may not be perceived by the patient at all, in which case it is called a *negative scotoma*. The lesion is usually in the optic nerve or retina but may occur anywhere from the retina to the occipital lobe.

In the history, is (are) there:
1. **Excessive tobacco use?** Tobacco poisoning may cause a scotoma, often bilaterally and centrally or paracentrally.
2. **Chronic alcoholism?** Methyl alcohol exposure, either intentionally or accidentally, may cause a scotoma or total blindness.
3. **Other members of the family affected?** Consider Leber's hereditary optic atrophy.
4. **Evidence that the scotoma is transient?** Consider migraine, transient ischemic attack, or multiple sclerosis.
5. **Loss of hair or other evidence of hormone deficiency?** Consider a pituitary tumor.

On physical examination, is (are) there:
1. **Increased intraocular pressure?** Consider glaucoma.
2. **Papilledema or papillitis?** Consider optic neuritis or brain tumor.
3. **Abnormalities on retinal examination?** Consider chorioretinitis, retinal detachment, or "eclipse" blindness.
4. **Hyperactive reflexes, sensory loss, or other neurologic findings?** Consider multiple sclerosis, space-occupying lesion, or cerebrovascular disease.

Diagnostic Workup
1. Ophthalmologic consultation
2. Visual field (multiple sclerosis)
3. Carotid sonography (carotid artery insufficiency)
4. Visual evoked potentials (multiple sclerosis)
5. Slit lamp examination (keratitis, iritis)
6. Pituitary function studies (pituitary tumor)
7. Tonometry (glaucoma)
8. Histamine test (migraine)
9. CT scan or MRI (brain tumor, multiple sclerosis)

SLEEP APNEA

In sleep apnea, respiration ceases or seems to cease for excessive periods while the patient is sleeping. The lesion may be located in the respiratory tree, obstructing ventilation (obstructive sleep apnea), or in the central nervous system, inhibiting the nervous impulse for respiration (central sleep apnea).

In the history, is there:
1. **Drug or alcohol use?** Drug and/or alcohol may suppress the respiratory center, causing central sleep apnea.
2. **Obesity?** Obesity is a common cause of both obstructive and central sleep apnea.
3. **Hypothyroidism or acromegaly?** Both conditions cause enlargement of the tongue or palate, leading to obstructive sleep apnea.
4. **Snoring?** Consider obstructive sleep apnea.
5. **Shortness of breath?** Consider congestive heart failure or emphysema.

On physical examination, is (are) there:
1. **Enlarged tonsils, palate, tongue, or nasal polyps?** These conditions may lead to obstructive sleep apnea.
2. **Sibilant and sonorous rales?** Chronic bronchitis and emphysema may cause obstructive sleep apnea.
3. **Pitting edema?** Consider congestive heart failure.
4. **Abnormal neurologic findings?** Consider poliomyelitis, Shy-Drager syndrome, brainstem tumor, or basilar artery insufficiency.

Diagnostic Workup
1. Complete blood count (anemia)
2. Arterial blood gases (emphysema, pulmonary fibrosis, congestive heart failure)
3. Spirometry (emphysema, pulmonary fibrosis)
4. Echocardiography (congestive heart failure)
5. Polysomnography (obstructive and central sleep apnea)
6. Otolaryngologic consultation
7. Pulmonologic consultation
8. Neurologic consultation

SLEEPWALKING

The definition of sleepwalking is self-evident. The cause is usually psychological, but a lesion may be located in the temporal lobe (complex partial seizures).

In the history, are there:
1. **Only rare episodes?** In this case, the sleepwalking is probably of no clinical significance.
2. **Additional psychological symptoms?** If the patient experiences bed-wetting, temper tantrums, or other psychological symptoms, sleepwalking may be a sign of a severe underlying psychological or social problem.
3. **Other signs of a seizure disorder?** Complex partial seizures (psychomotor epilepsy) may be associated with sleepwalking.

On physical examination, is (are) there:
1. **Lacerations of the tongue?** Consider the possibility of a seizure disorder.
2. **Multiple scars or bruises?** Look for child abuse.
3. **Factitious dermatitis?** Consider anxiety neurosis.

Diagnostic Workup
1. EEG, awake and asleep (epilepsy)
2. Psychometric testing (anxiety neurosis)
3. Psychiatric consultation
4. Neurologic consultation

SYNCOPE

Syncope is a transient loss of consciousness lasting only seconds to a few minutes. It is usually associated with impaired cerebral blood flow; consequently, the lesion is usually located in the cardiovascular system.

In the history, is (are) there:
1. **Drug use?** Many prescription drugs may lower blood pressure, leading to syncope. Beta-blockers, diuretics, ganglionic blockers, nitrates, and tranquilizers are just a few.
2. **Insulin-dependent diabetes?** Hypoglycemia may lead to syncope.
3. **Convulsive movements?** These suggest epilepsy (see page 10), although slightly convulsive movements may occur in common fainting spells.
4. **Chronic anxiety or depression?** Look for a psychogenic cause or hyperventilation syndrome.

On physical examination, is (are) there:
1. **Pallor?** Look for anemia or acute hemorrhage.
2. **Slow or absent pulse?** Look for heart block, vasovagal syncope, or carotid sinus syncope.
3. **Rapid pulse?** Consider supraventricular tachycardia, auricular fibrillation, ventricular tachycardia, heat exhaustion, or heat stroke.
4. **Heart murmur?** Consider syncope from aortic stenosis or insufficiency, or other valvular lesion of the heart.
5. **Focal neurologic signs?** Look for stroke, hypoglycemia, or transient ischemic attack (TIA).
6. **Profuse sweating?** Look for hypoglycemia or recent myocardial infarction.

Diagnostic Workup
1. Complete blood count (anemia)
2. Chemistry panel (hypoglycemia, etc.)
3. ECG (cardiac arrhythmia)
4. Urine drug screen (drug intoxication)
5. C-peptide analysis (hyperinsulinism)
6. 24-hour Holter monitoring (cardiac arrhythmia)
7. Echocardiography (valvular heart disease)
8. Carotid duplex scan (carotid stenosis)
9. EEG (seizure disorder)
10. 72-hour fast (insulinoma)
11. MRI of the brain (space-occupying lesion)
12. Four-vessel cerebral angiography or MRA (TIA)

TINNITUS

Tinnitus is a ringing, hissing, or roaring sound in one or both ears. The location of the lesion is usually the external middle or inner ear or the acoustic nerve, but it may occur in the brainstem or brain.

In the history, is (are) there:
1. **Unilateral involvement?** This would suggest neoplasm, infection, or trauma as the etiology. Bilateral involvement would suggest a degenerative or toxic etiology.
2. **Trauma?** Trauma to the ear or head may damage the middle or inner ear, causing tinnitus.
3. **Drug use?** Certain drugs, such as gentamicin, streptomycin, and kanamycin, may cause tinnitus. Aspirin, quinine, and the tricyclic antidepressants also may cause tinnitus.
4. **Occupational hazard?** Occupations that expose one to excessive noise may cause tinnitus.
5. **Pain in the ear?** Consider otitis externa or otitis media. A foreign body in the external canal may cause tinnitus.
6. **Headache?** Consider migraine or space-occupying lesion of the brain.
7. **Deafness with vertigo?** Consider Meniere's disease or acoustic neuroma.
8. **Deafness without vertigo?** Consider otosclerosis as the most likely cause; however, acoustic neuromas and Meniere's disease may occasionally present this way.

On physical examination, is (are) there:
1. **Abnormalities on examination of the ear?** Otoscopic examination may disclose a foreign body, wax, inflammation or perforation of the eardrum, mastoiditis, or cholesteatoma.
2. **Carotid bruit?** An atheroma of the carotid artery may be the source of the "tinnitus."
3. **Other cranial nerve signs?** Consider acoustic neuroma, multiple sclerosis, or early brainstem tumor.
4. **Long tract signs?** Consider multiple sclerosis, neurosyphilis, vertebral-basilar artery insufficiency, or advanced acoustic neuroma or brainstem tumor.

Diagnostic Workup
1. Complete blood count (anemia)
2. Sedimentation rate (infection)
3. Venereal Disease Research Laboratory (VDRL) test (neurosyphilis)
4. Thyroid profile (myxedema)
5. Radiography of the mastoid (mastoiditis)
6. Audiometry (otosclerosis, acoustic neuroma, Meniere's disease)
7. Caloric tests (acoustic neuroma, Meniere's disease)
8. Electronystagmography (Meniere's disease, acoustic neuroma)
9. MRI or CT scan (acoustic neuroma, brainstem tumor)
10. Spinal tap (multiple sclerosis, neurosyphilis)
11. Magnetic resonance angiography (vertebral-basilar artery insufficiency or aneurysm)
12. Four-vessel cerebral angiography (vertebral-basilar artery disease)

TRANSIENT ISCHEMIC ATTACK

A transient ischemic attack (TIA) is an attack of hemiplegia, monoplegia, or other neurologic deficit lasting less than 24 hours, and usually less than 30 minutes, with apparent complete clinical recovery. TIAs are almost always caused by brain or brainstem ischemia.

In the history, is (are) there:
1. **Headaches?** Consider migraine or seizures induced by a space-occupying lesion.
2. **Insulin-dependent diabetes?** Consider episodes of hypoglycemia. An insulinoma may cause similar attacks.
3. **Epilepsy?** Epileptic seizures may mimic a TIA.
4. **Chronic anxiety or depression?** Consider a conversion reaction.
5. **Heart disease?** Cardiac arrhythmias, myocardial infarction, and cardiomyopathy may be associated with TIA.

On physical examination, is there:
1. **Carotid bruit?** Consider carotid artery insufficiency.
2. **Diminished radial pulse?** Consider subclavian steal syndrome.
3. **Limitation of motion of the cervical spine?** Consider cervical spondylosis with compression of the vertebral arteries.
4. **Papilledema?** Consider a space-occupying lesion.
5. **Heart murmur?** Consider subacute bacterial endocarditis, mural thrombus, or atrial myxoma.
6. **Irregular heart rate?** Consider auricular fibrillation.

Diagnostic Workup
1. Complete blood count (anemia)
2. Chemistry panel (hypoglycemia)
3. Venereal Disease Research Laboratory (VDRL) test (neurosyphilis)
4. Chest radiography (metastatic neoplasm)
5. ECG (cardiac arrhythmia, myocardial infarction)
6. Carotid duplex scan (carotid artery stenosis)
7. Echocardiography (mural thrombus, atrial myxoma, etc.)
8. MRI and magnetic resonance angiography (brain tumor, vascular insufficiency)
9. EEG (epilepsy)
10. Four-vessel cerebral angiography (cerebrovascular disease)

WEAKNESS, GENERALIZED

The definition of weakness is self-evident. If the weakness is generalized, the lesion is usually located in the peripheral nerves, myoneural junction, or muscle. The cause may also be systemic.

In the history, is (are) there:
1. **Intermittent weakness?** This suggests myasthenia gravis or Eaton-Lambert syndrome.
2. **Drug or alcohol use or abuse?** A side effect of many prescription drugs is weakness or fatigue. Tranquilizers, beta-blockers, diuretics, and muscle relaxants are just a few agents with this side effect. Chronic alcoholism may produce weakness from a polyneuropathy, malnutrition, or an electrolyte imbalance.
3. **Overuse of caffeine or tobacco products?** These substances are well known to cause fatigue.
4. **Chronic anxiety or depression?** Many psychiatric disorders are associated with generalized weakness.
5. **Weight loss, polydipsia, and polyuria?** These symptoms should prompt consideration of diabetes mellitus, diabetes insipidus, hyperthyroidism, or hyperparathyroidism.
6. **Weight loss and polyphagia?** Consider diabetes mellitus or hyperthyroidism.
7. **Fever?** Consider septicemia, tuberculosis, infectious mononucleosis, or other systemic infection. Also consider lymphoma, leukemia, acquired immunodeficiency syndrome (AIDS), or metastatic neoplasm.
8. **Obesity?** Consider Cushing's syndrome.

On physical examination, is (are) there:
1. **Pallor?** Consider anemia, collagen disease, or neoplasm.
2. **Hypoactive reflexes and glove and stocking hypesthesia?** Consider polyneuropathy.
3. **Wasting of the muscles with preservation of reflexes?** Consider muscular dystrophy or dermatomyositis.
4. **Hyperactive reflexes?** Consider spinal cord or brainstem space-occupying lesion, primary lateral sclerosis, or multiple sclerosis.

Diagnostic Workup
1. Complete blood count (anemia, leukemia)
2. Sedimentation rate (systemic infection)
3. Chemistry panel (diabetes, uremia, liver disease)
4. Thyroid profile (hyperthyroidism)
5. Serum parathyroid hormone analysis (hyperparathyroidism)
6. Tensilon test (myasthenia gravis)
7. Acetylcholine receptor antibody analysis (myasthenia gravis)
8. Serum cortisol analysis (Addison's disease)
9. Febrile agglutinin analysis (infectious disease)
10. Monospot test (mononucleosis)
11. Serial blood cultures (septicemia, subacute bacterial endocarditis)
12. Human immunodeficiency disease antibody titer (AIDS)
13. Urine porphobilinogen analysis (porphyria)
14. Bone scan (metastatic malignancy, multiple myeloma)
15. Antinuclear antibody titer (collagen disease)
16. MRI of the brain and/or spinal cord (multiple sclerosis, tumor)
17. Drug screen (drug intoxication)
18. Infectious disease consultation
19. Oncologic consultation
20. Endocrinologic consultation
21. Muscle biopsy (muscular dystrophy, collagen disease)

WEAKNESS OF THE LOWER EXTREMITIES

The definition of lower extremity weakness is self-evident. The location of the lesion will usually be in the spinal cord, nerve roots, peripheral nerves, or muscle, but the lesion may occur in the parasagittal region of the brain or in the myoneural junctions.

In the history, is (are) there:
1. **Trauma?** Consider herniated disc, fracture of the spine, or contusion of the spinal cord.
2. **Intermittent claudication?** Consider peripheral arteriosclerosis, Leriche syndrome, or spinal stenosis.
3. **Pain in one or both of the lower extremities?** Consider herniated disc or cauda equina tumor.
4. **Incontinence?** Consider a space-occupying lesion of the spinal cord, multiple sclerosis, or trauma.
5. **Urinary retention?** Consider tabes dorsalis, diabetic neuropathy, or cauda equina tumor.

On physical examination, is (are) there:
1. **Cranial nerve involvement?** Consider a brainstem lesion or multiple sclerosis.
2. **Dermatomal sensory loss?** This suggests a herniated disc.
3. **Diffuse sensory loss?** Consider polyneuropathy or parasagittal tumor.
4. **Positive straight leg–raising test?** Consider herniated lumbar disc L4-L5 or L5-S1.
5. **Positive femoral stretch test?** Consider herniated disc of lumbar spine at L3-L4.
6. **Sensory level?** Consider spinal cord tumor.
7. **Diminished peripheral pulses?** Consider peripheral arteriosclerosis, Leriche syndrome, or femoral artery stenosis.

Diagnostic Workup
1. Complete blood count (pernicious anemia)
2. Venereal Disease Research Laboratory (VDRL) test (tabes dorsalis)
3. Glucose tolerance test (diabetic neuropathy)
4. Blood lead level (lead neuropathy)
5. Nerve conduction velocity studies (peripheral neuropathy, herniated disc)
6. Electromyography (herniated disc, muscular dystrophy)
7. MRI of the spine (herniated disc, tumor)
8. Somatosensory evoked potentials (multiple sclerosis)
9. Tensilon test (myasthenia gravis)
10. Muscle biopsy (muscular dystrophy)
11. Spinal tap (multiple sclerosis, neurosyphilis)

WEAKNESS OF THE UPPER EXTREMITIES

The definition of upper extremity weakness is self-evident. The lesion is located anywhere from the cerebral cortex to the brainstem; to the spinal cord, nerve roots, peripheral nerves, and myoneural junction; or to the muscles.

In the history is (are) there:
1. **Trauma?** Consider fracture of the spine, herniated disc, subdural or epidural hematoma, or contusion of the spinal cord or cerebrum.
2. **Pain in the extremity?** This would suggest a herniated cervical disc, fracture, or spinal cord tumor. If the pain and weakness are intermittent, consider coronary insufficiency or thoracic outlet syndrome.
3. **Transient attacks?** Consider carotid or basilar artery insufficiency, or subclavian steal syndrome. Also consider myasthenia gravis.
4. **Acute or gradual onset?** Acute onset suggests a neoplastic or degenerative lesion.

On physical examination, is (are) there:
1. **Cranial nerve signs?** Consider cerebrovascular disease, space-occupying lesion of the brain, or multiple sclerosis.
2. **Hyperactive reflexes of the involved extremity?** Consider stroke or tumor of the brain, brainstem, or spinal cord. Also consider multiple sclerosis.
3. **Hypoactive reflexes of the involved extremity?** Consider herniated disc, brachial plexus neuropathy, peripheral neuropathy, or ulnar or median nerve entrapment.
4. **Dermatomal sensory loss?** Consider herniated disc or other condition of the nerve roots.
5. **Tinel's sign of the wrist?** Consider carpal tunnel syndrome.
6. **Tinel's sign of the elbow?** Consider ulnar entrapment.
7. **Symmetric atrophy?** Consider muscular dystrophy.
8. **Asymmetric atrophy?** Consider amyotrophic lateral sclerosis, herniated disc, or syringomyelia.
9. **A sensory level?** Consider spinal cord tumor.
10. **Positive Adson's test?** Consider thoracic outlet syndrome.

Diagnostic Workup
1. Complete blood count (epidural abscess)
2. Sedimentation rate (epidural abscess)
3. Chemistry panel (neuropathy)
4. Venereal Disease Research Laboratory (VDRL) test (neurosyphilis)
5. ECG (coronary insufficiency, arrhythmia with embolism)
6. Radiography of the chest (Pancoast's tumor)
7. Radiography of the cervical spine (cervical rib, herniated disc, trauma)
8. MRI of the cervical spine or brain (tumor, multiple sclerosis, herniated disc, cerebrovascular disease)
9. Arteriography (cerebrovascular disease)
10. Nerve conduction velocity studies (carpal tunnel syndrome, ulnar entrapment)
11. Spinal fluid analysis (multiple sclerosis, neurosyphilis)
12. Electromyography (muscular dystrophy, muscular atrophy)
13. Tensilon test (myasthenia gravis)
14. Blood lead level (lead neuropathy)
15. Antinuclear antibody titers (collagen disease)

PART TWO

The Differential Diagnosis of Neurologic Signs

The Routine Neurologic Examination

Although you may already have an idea of how to perform a neurologic examination, you may be able to learn something from the way I do it.

In the office, I like to have the patient sitting on the examination table as comfortable as possible, with his or her legs dangling. In the hospital, I like to do the same thing, if possible, with the patient sitting on the side of the bed with his or her legs hanging over the edge. The room should be warm: neither freezing nor hot. The patient need not be fully undressed, but he or she should have shoes and socks removed.

I start by feeling the head for exostoses and listening for bruits over the eyes, head, and neck. This impresses the patient, and often gives him or her confidence that I know what I'm doing. Next, I look at the eye grounds (second cranial nerve). It is a good idea to dim the lights but not have them completely off, so the patient can look at a point or a thumb to fixate his or her eyes. I look primarily for optic atrophy or papilledema as well as hemorrhage or exudates. I check the response of the pupils to light and accommodation (second and third cranial nerves), then I check the visual fields (second cranial nerve) via confrontation with my fingers. If the patient complains of blindness or blurred vision, I do the visual field testing with a hat pin or cotton swab; I also prefer to stimulate all quadrants simultaneously. Next, I check the extraocular movements (third, fourth, and sixth cranial nerves) by having the patient follow my finger right and left and up and down with his or her eyes. These maneuvers also allow me to check for nystagmus (eighth cranial nerve and cerebellum). To check trochlear nerve function, I also have the patient look up and down while gazing to the left and then to the right. I then check the corneal reflex (fifth cranial nerve) with a cotton swab or horse hair. This can also be done by blowing gently on the eye. I use the cotton swab to check the sensation over the face; however, unless there is a complaint of facial numbness, I do not test for sensation to pain. Next, I check the facial muscles (seventh cranial nerve) by having the patient smile, grit his or her teeth, wrinkle his or her forehead, and close his or her eyes tightly.

To check the hearing (eighth cranial nerve), I rub my fingers close to each ear or whisper numbers into each ear. If the responses are abnormal, I perform a Weber or Rinne test (see Appendix A). To assess the ninth and tenth cranial nerves, I check the gag reflex with a cotton swab and have the patient swallow while I feel his or her Adam's apple, noting the quality of his or her voice at the same time. Next, I check the twelfth cranial nerve by having the patient stick out his or her tongue and move it side to side. Then, to check the eleventh cranial nerve, I ask the patient to shrug his or her shoulders and turn his or her head side to side while I apply pressure to his or her cheek with my hand. Next, I check the mobility of the neck laterally and on flexion and extension and rotation. This is important when the history suggests meningeal irritation or if a cervical spine disorder is suspected. In the latter case, I also perform a cervical compression test.

Now I get ready to check the extremities. I start by rapidly moving my hands, alternating left and right, while the patient slaps each hand with one of his or her hands. This movement tests the competency of the cerebellum and cerebellar tracts. Then, I have the patient touch his or her finger to his or her nose bilaterally while I look for any tremor at rest or on intention. To check the pyramidal tracts, motor nerves, and muscles, I ask the patient to squeeze my fingers, flex his or her biceps against resistance, and dorsiflex and plantarflex his or her feet and toes against resistance. If there is poor performance, I check more muscles in detail. Then, I take my reflex hammer and tap the biceps, triceps, and brachioradialis tendons in the upper extremities and the patellar and Achilles reflexes in the lower extremities. I stroke the bottom of the feet for a Babinski sign, and if I'm not satisfied with the response, I also look for Chaddock and Gordon signs. To evaluate the superficial abdominal reflexes (pyramidal tracts), I ask the patient to lie down, then I stroke his or her abdomen with the non–cotton-tipped end of a cotton swab.

Next, I do a sensory examination of the extremities. First, I check each extremity with the cotton swab for tactile sense (dorsal column, nerve roots, peripheral nerves), then I touch the swab to both upper then both lower extremities simultaneously to test for extinction, then I use a safety pin to prick the extremities (spinothalamic tracts, nerve roots, peripheral nerves). Finally, I check for vibratory sense with a 128 cps tuning fork and assess position sense by having the patient close his or her eyes and tell me the position of his or her thumb on each upper extremity and toe on each lower extremity. If the findings are equivocal, I draw numbers on the extremities while the patient closes his or her eyes and determines whether he or she can recognize the numbers.

In the final part of the examination, I ask the patient to stand and walk. If I detect any peculiarity, I have the patient walk on his or her heels and toes and then in tandem fashion (heel to toe). Then, I have the patient stand at ease while I check the sacrospinalis muscles for tension, an important step in patients with back pain. Finally, I perform a Romberg test by asking the patient to stand with feet close together and eyes closed. This test evaluates the integrity of the posterior columns, sensory nerve roots, and peripheral nerves.

I've just described my routine neurologic examination, which, in its entirety, takes less than a half hour. If I suspect dementia, I also perform a mental status examination (see Appendix A). If I suspect a lumbar herniated disc, I do straight leg–raising and femoral stretch tests. Other special examinations that may be employed are listed in Appendix A.

How do you record the neurologic examination in the chart? Here's a technique for a normal neurologic examination I learned years ago in my residency:

> The cranial nerves are intact, there is no papilledema or optic atrophy, and the pupils are equal and react to light and accommodations (PERLA). Visual fields are normal to confrontation, extraocular movements are intact, and there is no nystagmus. There is no facial, palatal, or lingual weakness. The extremities show good power, coordination, and sensation to all modalities on all four. Deep tendon reflexes are active and symmetric. There are no pathologic reflexes noted. Gait and station are intact.

The remainder of this section is devoted to the discussion of what each abnormality in the neurologic examination means, and its differential diagnosis. Under each neurologic sign, you will find additional things to look for in the history and examination.

ANKLE CLONUS

Ankle clonus is an alternating flexion and extension motion of the foot, which may be spontaneous or induced by rapidly dorsiflexing the foot and holding it in that position by slight pressure. The lesion is most likely in the pyramidal tract; however, the motion may be normal if it is bilateral and symmetric.

In the history, is (are) there:
1. **Complaints of weakness in one or more extremity?** Consider stroke, neoplasm of the brain or spinal cord, or multiple sclerosis.
2. **Recurrent left- or right-sided weakness?** Consider transient ischemic attack or multiple sclerosis.
3. **Fever or chills?** Consider brain abscess or epidural abscess of the spinal cord.
4. **Headaches?** Consider the possibility of cerebral hemorrhage or migraine.
5. **Previously diagnosed neoplasm of the lung, breast, or other organ?** Consider metastatic neoplasm of the brain or spinal cord.

On physical examination, is there:
1. **Unilateral clonus with cranial nerve signs?** Consider brain or brainstem space-occupying lesion or stroke.
2. **Unilateral clonus without cranial nerve signs?** Consider a spinal cord lesion such as multiple sclerosis, tumor, or amyotrophic lateral sclerosis. However, a parasagittal tumor may be the cause.
3. **Bilateral clonus with cranial nerve signs?** Consider brainstem tumor, syringomyelia, bulbar amyotrophic lateral sclerosis, syringobulbia, basilar artery disease, or multiple sclerosis.
4. **Bilateral clonus without cranial nerve signs?** Consider spinal cord tumor, multiple sclerosis, anterior spinal artery occlusion, or trauma.
5. **A sensory level?** Consider spinal cord tumor or syringomyelia.

Diagnostic Workup
1. CT scan or MRI of the brain (space-occupying lesion, cerebrovascular disease, multiple sclerosis)
2. MRI of the cervical or thoracic spinal cord (space-occupying lesion, anterior spinal artery occlusion, multiple sclerosis)
3. Spinal tap (multiple sclerosis, neurosyphilis)

APHASIA

Aphasia is the inability to receive, comprehend, or express words or sentences. The location of the lesion may be the temporal, parietal, or frontal lobe of the dominant hemisphere.

In the history, is (are) there:
1. **Sudden onset?** Consider cerebral embolism, thrombosis, or hemorrhage.
2. **Gradual onset?** Suspect a space-occupying lesion or degenerative disorder.
3. **Trauma?** Suspect an epidural, subdural, or intracerebral hematoma.
4. **Fever?** Look for encephalitis or brain abscess.
5. **Chronic alcoholism?** Look for Korsakoff's psychosis.
6. **Dementia?** Consider Alzheimer's disease, Creutzfeldt-Jakob disease, Pick's disease, herpes encephalitis, or Korsakoff's psychosis.
7. **Episodic attacks?** Consider transient ischemic attack, epilepsy, or migraine.

On physical examination, is there:
1. **Papilledema?** Suspect a space-occupying lesion of the brain.
2. **Hypertension?** Suspect a cerebral hemorrhage.
3. **Cardiac arrhythmia or murmur?** Consider the possibility of a cerebral embolism.

Diagnostic Workup
1. Venereal Disease Research Laboratory (VDRL) test (general paresis)
2. Blood alcohol level (Korsakoff's psychosis)
3. CT scan or MRI (space-occupying lesion, cerebrovascular disease)
4. EEG (epilepsy)
5. Spinal tap (neurosyphilis, encephalitis, multiple sclerosis)
6. Four-vessel cerebral angiography (cerebrovascular disease)
7. Neurologic consultation

ATAXIA

Ataxia is an uncoordinated gait. The lesion is typically located in the cerebellum, cerebellar tracts, or sensory tracts of the spinal cord and brainstem.

In the history, is (are) there:
1. **Vertigo, tinnitus, or deafness?** Consider acoustic neuroma, Meniere's disease, or multiple sclerosis.
2. **Secondary gain?** Consider hysteria or malingering.
3. **Headache?** Consider a brain tumor.
4. **Other members of the family affected?** Consider cerebellar ataxia.

On physical examination, is (are) there:
1. **Loss of vibratory and position senses in the lower extremities?** This would suggest pernicious anemia, Friedreich's ataxia, multiple sclerosis, advanced syringomyelia, or intramedullary tumor.
2. **No loss of vibratory and position sense?** Consider cerebellar tumor or degeneration. Drug or alcohol toxicity should also be considered.
3. **Cranial nerve signs?** Consider cerebellar or brainstem tumor, basilar artery disease, multiple sclerosis, or syringobulbia.
4. **Vertigo, tinnitus, or deafness?** Consider acoustic neuroma, Meniere's disease, or multiple sclerosis.
5. **Headaches, papilledema, or nystagmus?** Consider cerebellar tumor, hemorrhage, or acoustic neuroma.
6. **Positive Romberg test?** Consider a posterior column disease as in tabes dorsalis, pernicious anemia, Friedreich's ataxia, or multiple sclerosis. Also consider peripheral neuropathy.
7. **Secondary gain?** Consider hysteria or malingering.

Diagnostic Workup
1. Complete blood count (pernicious anemia)
2. Chemistry panel (diabetes)
3. Venereal Disease Research Laboratory (VDRL) test (tabes dorsalis)
4. Serum vitamin B_{12} analysis (pernicious anemia)
5. Audiogram and caloric tests (acoustic neuroma)
6. MRI of the spinal cord (spinal cord tumor, multiple sclerosis)
7. MRI of the brain (cerebellar tumor, acoustic neuroma, multiple sclerosis)
8. Spinal tap (multiple sclerosis, neurosyphilis, vascular disease)
9. Evoked potential studies (multiple sclerosis)
10. Four-vessel cerebral angiography (vertebral-basilar artery disease).

ATHETOSIS

Athetosis is the spontaneous writhing, smooth, sinuous movement of the hands and fingers or, less commonly, the face or feet. The lesion is usually in the basal ganglia.

In the history, is there:
1. **Onset at birth?** This would suggest cerebral palsy or kernicterus from erythroblastosis fetalis.
2. **Onset following a febrile illness?** Consider dystonia musculorum deformans or encephalitis.
3. **Onset in childhood or adulthood?** Consider Wilson's disease, Parkinson's disease, or postencephalitic parkinsonism.

On physical examination, is there:
1. **Tremor and/or rigidity?** This suggests a diagnosis of Parkinson's disease.
2. **Kayser-Fleischer ring?** Consider the possibility of Wilson's disease.

Diagnostic Workup
1. Chemistry panel (Wilson's disease)
2. Serum copper and ceruloplasmin analysis (Wilson's disease)
3. Heavy metal screen (manganese toxicity)
4. MRI (cerebral infarction, brain tumor)
5. Liver biopsy (Wilson's disease)

BABINSKI'S SIGN AND OTHER PATHOLOGIC REFLEXES

Babinski's sign is the dorsiflexion of the big toe and fanning of the other toes in response to stroking the outer border of the bottom of the foot from heel to toe. Other pathologic reflexes include Hoffmann's, Gordon's, Oppenheim, and Chaddock's reflexes, which have the same clinical significance (see Glossary). The lesion may be located anywhere along the pyramidal tract, from the cortex to the spinal cord. The lesion causing Hoffmann's reflex is found in the upper extremities.

In the history, is there:
1. **Trauma?** If there is head trauma, consider epidural or subdural hematoma. If there is trauma to the neck or back, consider the possibility of hematoma, contusion, or fracture of the spine with spinal cord compression.
2. **Headache?** This would suggest a space-occupying lesion of the brain.
3. **Pain in the extremities?** Look for spinal cord tumor, herniated disc of the cervical spine, epidural abscess or hematoma, and cervical spondylosis. A thalamic syndrome may need to be considered.
4. **Fever?** Suspect encephalitis, cerebral abscess, epidural abscess of the spinal cord, or stroke.
5. **Coma?** Consider encephalitis, cerebral hemorrhage, meningitis, abscess, drug or alcohol intoxication, or head injury. The pathologic reflexes cannot be used to localize the lesion when there is coma.

On physical examination, is (are) there:
1. **Hemiplegia?** Consider cerebrovascular disease or space-occupying lesion of the brain.
2. **Paraplegia without cranial nerve signs?** This suggests a lesion of the spinal cord, but remember, parasagittal lesions may present with this picture.
3. **Paraplegia with cranial nerve signs?** This suggests a brainstem lesion.
4. **A sensory level?** Consider spinal cord tumor or syringomyelia.
5. **Hypoactive reflexes of the involved extremity or extremities?** If there is recent trauma or stroke, hypoactive reflexes are to be expected. However, if the onset has been more insidious, suspect Friedreich's ataxia or pernicious anemia.

Diagnostic Workup
1. Complete blood count (infection, pernicious anemia)
2. Sedimentation rate (infection)
3. Venereal Disease Research Laboratory (VDRL) test (neurosyphilis)
4. MRI of the spinal cord (neoplasm, transverse myelitis, multiple sclerosis)
5. CT scan or MRI of the brain (space-occupying lesion, stroke, multiple sclerosis, degenerative disease)
6. Plain film of the skull or spine (trauma, metastatic neoplasm)
7. Carotid duplex scan (carotid stenosis)
8. Four-vessel cerebral angiography (cerebrovascular disease)
9. Neurologic consultation

CERVICAL BRUIT

Cervical bruit is a swishing sound or murmur picked up by the stethoscope when it is placed over the patient's neck. The lesion may be in the arteries, veins, or thyroid, or may be transmitted from the heart or aorta.

In the history, is (are) there:
1. **Sweating or heat intolerance?** Suspect hyperthyroidism.
2. **Episodes of transient hemiplegia?** Consider carotid stenosis or subclavian steal syndrome.
3. **Amaurosis fugax?** Consider carotid stenosis.

On physical examination, is (are) there:
1. **Pallor?** Consider anemia.
2. **Heart murmur?** Consider valvular heart disease.
3. **Enlarged thyroid?** Consider hyperthyroidism.
4. **Long tract neurologic signs?** Consider carotid stenosis or subclavian steal syndrome.
5. **Diminished radial pulse on the side of the bruit?** Consider subclavian steal syndrome.

Diagnostic Workup
1. Complete blood count (anemia)
2. Thyroid profile (hyperthyroidism)
3. Carotid duplex scan (carotid stenosis)
4. Angiography (carotid stenosis, subclavian steal)
5. Echocardiography (valvular heart disease)

CHOREA

Chorea is the occurrence of involuntary sudden, wild, jerky movements, often of the whole extremity, which are usually absent when the patient is relaxed. The lesion is located in the basal ganglia.

In the history, is (are) there:
1. **Early age of onset?** Consider Sydenham's chorea, Lesch-Nyhan syndrome, Wilson's disease, or Tourette's syndrome.
2. **Late age of onset?** Consider Huntington's chorea or senile chorea.
3. **A family history?** Consider Wilson's disease, Huntington's chorea, or Tourette' s syndrome.
4. **Fever and joint pain?** Consider Sydenham's chorea or encephalitis.
5. **Mental deficiency and delusions?** Consider Huntington's chorea.
6. **Drug ingestion?** Consider intoxication or sensitivity to phenothiazines, levodopa, anticonvulsants, or birth control pills.

On physical examination, is there:
1. **Kayser-Fleischer ring?** Consider Wilson's disease.

Diagnostic Workup
1. Sedimentation rate, antistreptolysin O titer (rheumatic fever)
2. Serum copper and ceruloplasmin (Wilson's disease)
3. Antinuclear antibody titer (lupus cerebritis)
4. Human immunodeficiency virus antibody titer (acquired immunodeficiency syndrome)
5. Neurologic consultation
6. MRI of the brain (Huntington's chorea)
7. Genetic testing

CONSTRICTED PUPIL

A constricted pupil is less than 3 mm in diameter. The lesion may be in the eye, the sympathetic pathways, or the midbrain.

In the history, is (are) there:
1. **Eye pain or blurred vision?** Consider iritis or uveitis.
2. **Headaches?** Consider migraine.
3. **Use of drugs?** Narcotics may cause constricted pupils.
4. **Coma?** Bilateral constricted pupils with coma may signal a brainstem hemorrhage.
5. **Dementia?** Consider general paresis.
6. **Pain in the neck or arm on the side of the lesion?** Consider thoracic outlet syndrome.

On physical examination, is (are) there:
1. **Poor response to light but good response to accommodation or convergence?** Consider the Argyll Robertson pupil of neurosyphilis or diabetes.
2. **Partial ptosis and enophthalmos?** Suspect Horner's syndrome (see page 67).

Diagnostic Workup
1. Venereal Disease Research Laboratory (VDRL) test (neurosyphilis)
2. Slit lamp examination (iritis)
3. Ophthalmologic consultation
4. Workup for Horner's syndrome (see page 67)
5. Urine drug screen (drug intoxication)
6. MRI (brainstem hemorrhage or tumor)
7. Spinal tap (neurosyphilis)

DILATED PUPIL

The normal pupil measures 3 to 4 mm. A dilated pupil is 5 mm or larger. The lesion may be located in the retina, optic nerve, or oculomotor nerve.

In the history, is there:
1. **Blindness?** Obviously, if the patient is blind in both eyes, the pupils will be dilated and unresponsive to light. However, if the blindness is restricted to one eye, the pupils will appear normal and will only dilate when the good eye is covered. The dilated pupil then responds when light is supplied to the good eye again (consensual response). The causes of blindness are covered on page 7.
2. **Drug use?** Narcotics, barbiturates, and anticholinergic drugs may cause dilated pupils.
3. **Trauma?** Consider epidural or subdural hematoma when there is a unilateral dilated pupil. A concussion may cause bilateral dilated pupils.
4. **Eye pain?** Suspect Wernicke's encephalopathy or methyl alcohol poisoning. However, the pupils usually do not become dilated until late in Wernicke's encephalopathy.
5. **Alcoholism?** Suspect Wernicke's encephalopathy or methyl alcohol poisoning. However, the pupils usually do not become dilated until late in Wernicke's encephalopathy.
6. **Headache?** Consider migraine, temporal arteritis, or a brain tumor.

On physical examination, is there:
1. **Paralysis of extraocular muscles supplied by the oculomotor nerve but no long tract signs?** Consider aneurysm of the circle of Willis.
2. **Paralysis of extraocular muscles supplied by the oculomotor nerve with long tract signs?** Consider brainstem infarct or space-occupying lesion.
3. **A response of the dilated pupil to light and accommodation?** This would suggest the problem is glaucoma, iritis, or anisocoria.
4. **Poor response of the dilated pupil to light and accommodation, but no other neurologic findings other than hypoactive reflexes?** Consider the possibility of Adie's syndrome.

Diagnostic Workup
1. Venereal Disease Research Laboratory (VDRL) test (neurosyphilis)
2. Sedimentation rate (temporal arteritis)
3. Visual field examination (optic neuritis, optic nerve lesions)
4. Tonometry (glaucoma)
5. Glucose tolerance test (diabetic neuropathy)
6. Response to intravenous thiamine (Wernicke's encephalopathy)
7. MRI (aneurysm, space-occupying lesion)
8. Angiography (aneurysm, cerebrovascular disease)

DYSARTHRIA

Dysarthria is difficulty in pronouncing words or slurring of the speech. The lesion is usually located in the brain or brainstem, but it may be in the myoneural junctions or muscle.

In the history, is there:
1. **Sudden onset?** This would suggest a cerebral embolism, thrombosis, or hemorrhage.
2. **Gradual onset?** Suspect a space-occupying lesion of the brain or brainstem, a degenerative disorder, or multiple sclerosis.
3. **Episodic occurrence?** This would suggest myasthenia gravis, epilepsy, or transient ischemic attack (TIA).
4. **Drug or alcohol use?** Alcohol and many drugs may cause slurred speech.
5. **Trauma?** Consider the possibility of concussion or subdural hematoma.

On physical examination, is there:
1. **Hemiplegia?** Consider cerebrovascular disease, tumor, or multiple sclerosis.
2. **Papilledema?** This would indicate a space-occupying lesion of the brain.
3. **Ataxia or nystagmus?** Look for drug or alcohol intoxication, cerebellar tumor, hereditary cerebellar ataxia, or multiple sclerosis.
4. **Tremor or rigidity?** Suspect Parkinson's disease or other extrapyramidal disorder.
5. **Atrophy of the muscles of the face and extremities?** Look for bulbar amyotrophic lateral sclerosis or muscular dystrophy.

Diagnostic Workup
1. Blood alcohol level (alcoholism)
2. Urine drug screen (drug intoxication)
3. Acetylcholine receptor antibody titer (myasthenia gravis)
4. Tensilon test (myasthenia gravis)
5. CT scan or MRI (space-occupying lesion, stroke, multiple sclerosis, degenerative disease)
6. EEG (seizure disorder)
7. Carotid duplex scan (TIA, stroke)
8. Serum copper and ceruloplasmin (Wilson's disease)
9. Spinal tap (neurosyphilis, multiple sclerosis)

EXOPHTHALMOS

Exophthalmos is a protrusion of the eyeballs. The lesion may be in the sinuses, orbit, vasculature, or pituitary or thyroid gland.

In the history, is there:
1. **Fever?** Consider orbital cellulitis, sinusitis, or cavernous sinus thrombosis.
2. **Trauma?** Consider orbital hemorrhage, traumatic arteriovenous aneurysm, fracture of the orbit, or orbital emphysema.
3. **Nasal discharge?** Consider sinusitis.

On physical examination, is there:
1. **Enlarged thyroid, tremor, or tachycardia?** Consider Graves' disease.
2. **Pulsation of the eyeball or an orbital bruit?** Consider arteriovenous aneurysm.
3. **Chemosis and ecchymosis?** Consider cavernous sinus thrombosis.

Diagnostic Workup
1. Complete blood count and sedimentation rate (orbital cellulitis, cavernous sinus thrombosis)
2. Thyroid profile (Graves' disease)
3. Radiography of the orbits (orbital cellulitis, tumor)
4. Radiography of the sinuses (sinusitis)
5. CT scan or MRI (orbital tumor, cavernous sinus thrombosis)
6. Angiography (arteriovenous aneurysm)
7. Thyrotropin receptor antibody concentration (pituitary exophthalmos)
8. Endocrinologic consultation

FACIAL PARALYSIS

Facial paralysis may be unilateral or bilateral. If the muscles of the forehead and orbit are spared, the lesion is probably central (involving the upper motor neurons). If all the facial muscles are involved, the lesion is in the peripheral nerve, myoneural junction, or muscle.

In the history, is there:
1. **Trauma?** Consider epidural or subdural hematoma or basilar skull fracture.
2. **Fever?** Consider petrositis, mastoiditis, poliomyelitis, or basilar meningitis.
3. **Symmetric involvement of the face and extremities?** Consider Guillain-Barré syndrome.
4. **Evidence of intermittent paralysis?** Consider myasthenia gravis or transient ischemic attack.
5. **Diabetes?** Consider diabetic neuropathy.

On physical examination, is (are) there:
1. **Papilledema?** Consider a space-occupying lesion.
2. **Rash of the external ear canal?** Consider Ramsay Hunt syndrome.
3. **Hemiplegia?** Consider cerebrovascular disease or a space-occupying lesion of the brain.
4. **Hearing loss?** Consider mastoiditis, petrositis, acoustic neuroma, or cholesteatoma.
5. **Premature baldness or corneal opacities?** Consider myotonic dystrophy.
6. **Horner's syndrome and crossed hemianalgesia of the face and extremities?** Consider posterior inferior cerebellar artery occlusion.

Diagnostic Workup
1. Complete blood count (middle ear infection, petrositis, brain abscess)
2. Venereal Disease Research Laboratory (VDRL) test (neurosyphilis)
3. Angiography and caloric tests (acoustic neuroma)
4. CT scan or MRI (brain tumor, cerebrovascular disease, multiple sclerosis)
5. Blood lead level (lead neuropathy)
6. Glucose tolerance test (diabetes mellitus)
7. Spinal tap (Guillain-Barré syndrome)
8. Lyme disease antibody titer (Lyme disease)
9. Electromyography (Bell's palsy)
10. Acetylcholine receptor antibody titer (myasthenia gravis)
11. Muscle biopsy (myotonic dystrophy)

FASCICULATIONS

Fasciculations are visible but tiny, spontaneous contractions of a portion of a muscle that usually are not strong enough to move the extremity or body part in which they occur. The lesion is usually located in the anterior horn cells of the spinal cord or motor root.

In the history, is (are) there:
1. **Neck or back pain?** Consider a herniated disc or other space-occupying lesion.
2. **Fever?** Consider the possibility of poliomyelitis or encephalomyelitis.
3. **Exposure to pesticides?** Look for organophosphate or carbamate poisoning.
4. **Focal fasciculations with pain?** Consider a spinal cord tumor or other space-occupying lesion.
5. **Focal fasciculations without pain?** Consider amyotrophic lateral sclerosis.
6. **Generalized fasciculations?** Look for Guillain-Barré syndrome or pesticide poisoning.

On physical examination, is there:
1. **A sensory level?** Look for spinal cord tumor or syringomyelia.
2. **Significant atrophy in the extremity where the fasciculations occur?** Consider amyotrophic lateral sclerosis or syringomyelia. A spinal cord tumor is less likely.
3. **Symmetric atrophy of the lower extremities?** Look for peroneal muscular atrophy.

Diagnostic Workup
1. Complete blood count and chemistry panel (toxic neuropathy or pesticide poisoning)
2. MRI (spinal cord tumor, herniated disc, syringomyelia)
3. Electromyography (amyotrophic lateral sclerosis)
4. Spinal tap (Guillian-Barré syndrome, poliomyelitis)
5. Nerve conduction velocity study (neuropathy)

GAIT DISTURBANCE

Gait disturbance is simply difficulty in walking. The lesion may be anywhere along the motor, sensory, or cerebellar tracts from the brain to the spinal cord, nerve roots, peripheral nerves, and muscles. It may also occur in the bones and joints.

In the history, is (are) there:
1. **Malnutrition?** Consider peripheral neuropathy.
2. **Other family members affected?** Look for cerebellar ataxia or muscular dystrophy.
3. **Back pain?** Look for spinal cord tumor.
4. **Vertigo?** Consider Meniere's disease.
5. **Diabetes?** Consider diabetic neuropathy.

On physical examination, is there:
1. **A limp?** If the patient limps, he or she is favoring one extremity over the other because of pain or stiffness in the involved extremity. Look for bone or joint inflammation or injury. Also look for contusion or inflammation of the muscle or soft tissue.
2. **A short-stepped gait?** This is the gait of Parkinson's disease and bilateral pyramidal tract involvement.
3. **A wide-based gait?** Look for cerebellar involvement (as in multiple sclerosis) or posterior column disease (as in tabes dorsalis or pernicious anemia).
4. **Weaving?** Look for cerebellar or posterior column involvement.
5. **A high-stepping gait?** A bilateral high-stepping gait is typical of peripheral neuropathy or a cauda equina lesion. A unilateral high-stepping gait indicates an L5 radiculopathy or neuropathy of the common peroneal nerve.
6. **A clownish gait with associated choreiform movements?** Consider Huntington's chorea.
7. **A pelvic tilt?** This would suggest muscular dystrophy.
8. **Deviation to one side while walking?** This is typical of a labyrinthine disturbance such as Meniere's disease but may also occur in tumors or other lesions of the cerebellar lobes.
9. **A consistent pattern to the gait?** Consider hysteria or malingering.

Diagnostic Workup
1. Complete blood count (pernicious anemia)
2. Serum vitamin B_{12} level (pernicious anemia)
3. Venereal Disease Research Laboratory (VDRL) test (tabes dorsalis)
4. Neuropathy workup (see page 167)
5. MRI of the brain (space-occupying lesion, multiple sclerosis, stroke)
6. MRI of the spinal cord (space-occupying lesion, multiple sclerosis, degenerative disease)
7. Electromyography (muscular dystrophy)
8. Muscle biopsy (muscular dystrophy)

HEMIANOPSIA

Hemianopsia is the loss of vision in one-half of the visual field of one or both eyes. If the hemianopsia is bilateral, it may be *homonymous*, in which case it involves the nasal field of one eye and the temporal field of the other, or it may be *bitemporal*, in which case it involves the temporal field of both eyes. It is rare for the hemianopsia to involve the nasal field of both eyes. If the field deficit involves only one quadrant of the field, it is called a *quadrantanopsia*. The hemianopsia may be incomplete and may not involve the central portion of the visual field, in which case it is called *hemianopsia with macular sparing*. The location of the lesion may be the retina, optic nerve, optic chiasma, optic tract, optic radiation, or occipital cortex.

In the history, is there:
1. **Intermittent occurrence?** This suggests migraine or transient ischemic attack.
2. **Sudden onset?** This suggests a cerebral embolism, thrombosis, or hemorrhage, but it might also indicate a cerebral aneurysm or multiple sclerosis.
3. **Gradual onset?** This suggests glaucoma or a space-occupying lesion of the brain or brainstem.
4. **Trauma?** Consider damage to the optic nerve or chiasm, brainstem hematoma, or subdural hematoma compressing the occipital cortex or optic radiations.
5. **Fever?** Consider cortical abscess, collagen disease, or tuberculoma.

On physical examination, is there:
1. **Increased extraocular pressure?** Consider glaucoma or vitreous hemorrhage.
2. **Bitemporal hemianopsia?** Consider a pituitary tumor or aneurysm compressing the optic chiasm.
3. **Homonymous hemianopsia?** Consider a space-occupying lesion or stroke involving the brainstem or occipital cortex.
4. **Quadrantanopsia?** Consider a space-occupying lesion of the temporal lobe.
5. **Macular sparing?** This suggests a space-occupying lesion of the occipital cortex or posterior cerebral artery occlusion.
6. **Hemiplegia or hemianesthesia?** This suggests a space-occupying lesion of the brain, middle cerebral artery or basilar artery occlusion, or multiple sclerosis.

Diagnostic Workup
1. Ophthalmologic consultation
2. CT scan or MRI (space-occupying lesion, cerebrovascular disease)
3. Venereal Disease Research Laboratory (VDRL) test (neurosyphilis)
4. Antinuclear antibody titer (collagen disease)
5. Carotid duplex scan (carotid artery stenosis)
6. Magnetic resonance angiography (aneurysm, cerebrovascular disease)
7. Four-vessel cerebral angiography (vertebral-basilar or carotid artery insufficiency)
8. Spinal tap (multiple sclerosis, neurosyphilis)
9. ECG (cardiac arrhythmia)
10. Cardiologic consultation
11. Endocrinologic consultation (pituitary tumor)

HEMIPARESIS/HEMIPLEGIA

Hemiparesis is weakness or partial paralysis, and hemiplegia is complete paralysis, of the arm and leg on one side of the body. The lesion is usually somewhere along the pyramidal tract, from the cervical spine to the cerebral cortex. Poliomyelitis and mononeuritis multiplex occasionally may simulate hemiplegia.

In the history, is there:
1. **Intermittent occurrence?** Consider migraine, multiple sclerosis, or transient ischemic attack.
2. **Sudden onset?** This would suggest a cerebral embolism, hemorrhage, or thrombosis, unless the hemiplegia or hemiparesis follows trauma. In that case, it is more likely caused by an epidural or subdural hematoma.
3. **Gradual onset?** This would suggest a space-occupying lesion of the brain or cervical spinal cord.
4. **Trauma?** Consider epidural, subdural, or intracerebral hematoma. Also consider spinal cord contusion, although this is more likely to present with paraplegia or quadriplegia.
5. **Fever?** Consider cerebral abscess or subacute bacterial endocarditis (SBE).

On physical examination, is (are) there:
1. **Central facial paralysis or other cranial nerve signs?** If so, consider a space-occupying lesion or stroke of the brain or brainstem. If not, consider a lesion of the cervical spinal cord.
2. **Hypertension?** Consider cerebral hemorrhage. However, ischemic infarcts and cerebral aneurysms may be associated with a history of hypertension.
3. **Coma?** Consider cerebral hemorrhage or aneurysm.
4. **Cardiac murmur or arrhythmia?** Consider cerebral embolism or SBE.
5. **Carotid bruit?** Consider carotid stenosis or thrombosis.

Diagnostic Workup
1. Complete blood count and sedimentation rate (cerebral abscess)
2. Antinuclear antibody titer (collagen disease)
3. Venereal Disease Research Laboratory (VDRL) test (neurosyphilis)
4. Blood cultures (SBE)
5. ECG (cardiac arrhythmia, myocardial infarction)
6. Carotid duplex scan (carotid artery stenosis)
7. MRI of the spinal cord (space-occupying lesion, cerebrovascular disease)
8. CT scan (cerebral hemorrhage)
9. Magnetic resonance angiography (cerebrovascular disease, aneurysm)
10. Echocardiography (mural thrombosis)
11. Spinal fluid analysis (multiple sclerosis, neurosyphilis)

HORNER SYNDROME

Horner syndrome is the combination of miosis, partial ptosis, and enophthalmos. The lesion may be anywhere along the sympathetic pathway, from the brainstem to the spinal cord, to the chest, to the neck, or to the orbit.

In the history, is (are) there:
1. **Headaches?** Consider migraine or histamine headaches.
2. **Pain in the neck and upper extremity?** Consider cervical rib, scalenus anticus syndrome, Pancoast's tumor, Hodgkin's disease, or brachial plexus injury.

On physical examination, is (are) there:
1. **A bruit over the carotid artery?** Consider carotid stenosis or thrombosis.
2. **A mass in the neck?** Consider Hodgkin's disease or Pancoast's tumor.
3. **Hemiplegia?** This suggests carotid thrombosis.
4. **Long tract signs in the extremities without cranial nerve signs?** Consider a spinal cord lesion such as syringomyelia, tumor, myeloma, or neurosyphilis.
5. **Long tract signs with evidence of cranial nerve involvement?** Consider a brainstem glioma, syringobulbia, encephalitis, or posterior inferior cerebellar artery occlusion.

Diagnostic Workup
1. Carotid duplex scan (carotid artery thrombosis)
2. Radiography of the cervical spine (cervical rib)
3. Radiography of the chest (Pancoast's tumor)
4. CT scan of the mediastinum (mediastinal tumor)
5. MRI of the cervical spinal cord (tumor, syringomyelia)
6. MRI of the brain (brainstem glioma, Wallenberg syndrome)
7. Nerve conduction velocity studies and somatosensory evoked potentials (brachial plexus neuralgia)

HYPERACTIVE REFLEXES

Hyperactive reflexes are an increase in the deep tendon reflexes. If there is a symmetric increase in the deep tendon reflexes, it may be physiologic, but when there is an asymmetric increase, it is almost always pathologic. The lesion may be located anywhere along the pyramidal tract, from the brain to the spinal cord.

In the history, is there:
1. **Head trauma?** Hyperactive reflexes on one side of the body may indicate an epidural or subdural hematoma.
2. **Trauma to the spine?** Hyperactive reflexes of all four extremities may indicate a spinal cord contusion or epidural hematoma in the cervical spine, whereas hyperactive reflexes of only the lower extremities may indicate hematoma or contusion of the thoracic spinal cord. However, during the acute stages of such trauma, the reflexes would be depressed.
3. **Fever?** Fever with hyperactive reflexes on one side of the body suggests cerebral abscess, whereas fever with hyperactive reflexes of the lower extremities may indicate an epidural abscess of the spinal cord.
4. **Headache?** Headache with hyperactive reflexes of one side of the body may indicate a space-occupying lesion of the contralateral cerebral hemisphere.
5. **Radicular pain?** Radicular pain with hyperactive reflexes on the lower extremities suggests a space-occupying lesion of the spinal cord.
6. **Incontinence?** Consider a spinal cord lesion.

On physical examination, is (are) there:
1. **Papilledema?** Consider a space-occupying lesion of the brain or brainstem.
2. **Cranial nerve signs?** Consider a space-occupying lesion of the brain or brainstem, cerebrovascular disease, encephalitis, or multiple sclerosis.
3. **Unilateral dilated pupil?** Consider a space-occupying lesion of the brain.
4. **No cranial nerve signs or papilledema?** Consider a spinal cord lesion.
5. **A sensory level?** Consider a space-occupying lesion of the spinal cord.
6. **Dementia?** Suspect Alzheimer's disease, cerebral arteriosclerosis, or general paresis.
7. **Ataxia and symmetric loss of vibratory and position senses?** Consider the possibility of pernicious anemia or Friedreich's ataxia.

Diagnostic Workup
1. Complete blood count (pernicious anemia)
2. Serum vitamin B_{12} level (pernicious anemia)
3. Venereal Disease Research Laboratory (VDRL) test (neurosyphilis)
4. CT scan or MRI of the brain (space-occupying lesion of the brain, stroke, multiple sclerosis)
5. MRI of the spine (tumor, multiple sclerosis)
6. Spinal tap (multiple sclerosis)
7. Somatosensory evoked potentials (multiple sclerosis)
8. Carotid duplex scan (carotid stenosis)
9. Four-vessel cerebral angiography (cerebrovascular disease)

HYPERKINESIA

Hyperkinesia is increased muscle activity, or increased activity of the body in general. The lesion is usually in the extrapyramidal system.

In the history, is (are) there:
1. **Drug use?** Prescription drugs such as phenothiazine, tricyclic antidepressants, and lithium may cause hyperkinesis. Cocaine and amphetamines are illegal drugs to be considered.
2. **Mental deficiency?** Consider Huntington's chorea or Wilson's disease.
3. **Fever and joint pain?** Consider Sydenham's chorea.

On physical examination, is (are) there:
1. **Tremor?** Consider Wilson's disease, hyperthyroidism, and Parkinson's disease.
2. **Goiter or tachycardia?** Consider hyperthyroidism.
3. **Chorea?** Consider Wilson's disease, Sydenham's chorea, or Huntington's chorea.
4. **Kayser-Fleischer ring?** Consider Wilson's disease.
5. **Absence of neurologic signs?** Consider attention deficit disorder, hyperthyroidism, or Tourette's syndrome.

Diagnosis Workup
1. Thyroid profile (hyperthyroidism)
2. Complete blood count, sedimentation rate, and antistreptolysin O titer (Sydenham's chorea)
3. Serum copper and ceruloplasmin (Wilson's disease)
4. Neurologic consultation
5. MRI of the brain (Huntington's chorea)
6. Psychiatric consultation

HYPOACTIVE REFLEXES

Hypoactive reflexes are decreased deep tendon reflexes. A symmetric decrease in deep tendon reflexes may be physiologic, but an asymmetric decrease in reflexes is usually pathologic. The lesion may be located in the anterior horn of the spinal cord, nerve roots, peripheral nerve, myoneural junction, or muscles.

In the history, is there:
1. **Trauma?** Recent head trauma may cause an epidural, subdural, or intracerebral hematoma, resulting in contralateral hypoactive reflexes in the acute stage. Recent spinal cord trauma may cause concussion, hemorrhage, or transection, leading to hypoactive reflexes of all extremities in the acute stage.
2. **Fever?** Diffuse hypoactive reflexes and fever bring to mind the possibility of Guillain-Barré syndrome, poliomyelitis, or spinal cord trauma.
3. **Acute onset?** Acute onset of hypoactive reflexes with weakness would suggest Guillain-Barré syndrome, poliomyelitis, or spinal cord trauma.
4. **Urinary retention or difficulty voiding?** Hypoactive reflexes in the lower extremities along with urinary retention would suggest a cauda equina lesion.
5. **Radiculopathy?** Consider herniated disc or other lesion of the nerve root.

On physical examination, (is) are there:
1. **Hemiplegia?** Consider a space-occupying lesion of the brain or cerebrovascular disease.
2. **Quadriplegia or paraplegia?** Consider a spinal cord lesion.
3. **Symmetric loss of vibratory and position senses?** Consider pernicious anemia, tabes dorsalis, or Friedreich's ataxia.
4. **Glove and stocking hypesthesia and hypalgesia?** Consider peripheral neuropathy.
5. **Dermatomal sensory loss?** Consider herniated disc or other disease of the nerve root.
6. **Diffuse fasciculations?** Consider progressive muscular atrophy.
7. **Proximal muscle wasting and a pelvic tilt?** Consider muscular dystrophy.

Diagnostic Workup
1. Complete blood count (pernicious anemia)
2. Serum vitamin B_{12} level (pernicious anemia)
3. Venereal Disease Research Laboratory (VDRL) test (tabes dorsalis)
4. Antinuclear antibody titer (collagen disease, dermatomyositis)
5. Glucose tolerance test (diabetic neuropathy)
6. CT scan or MRI of the brain (space-occupying lesion, cerebrovascular disease)
7. MRI of the spine (space-occupying lesion of the spine, herniated disc, spinal cord trauma).
8. Spinal tap (Guillain-Barré syndrome, poliomyelitis, tabes dorsalis)
9. Electromyography and nerve conduction velocity study (radiculopathy, muscular dystrophy)
10. Acetylcholine receptor antibody titer (myasthenia gravis)
11. Muscle biopsy (muscular dystrophy)

INTRACRANIAL BRUIT

An intracranial bruit is a murmur or swishing sound heard over the orbit or other areas of the skull. The lesion is usually in the arteries.

In the history, is (are) there:
1. **Malnutrition?** Consider nutritional anemia.
2. **Transient ischemic attacks?** Look for carotid insufficiency.
3. **Seizures?** Consider the possibility of an arteriovenous fistula.

On physical examination, is there:
1. **Pallor?** Suspect anemia.
2. **Proptosis?** Consider an arteriovenous fistula.
3. **A cervical bruit?** Consider carotid stenosis.

Diagnostic Workup
1. Complete blood count (anemia)
2. Carotid duplex scan (carotid stenosis)
3. MRI of the brain (angioma, aneurysm, arteriovenous fistula)
4. Angiography (aneurysm, angioma, arteriovenous fistula)

MUSCLE ATROPHY

Muscle atrophy is a decrease in the size of individual muscles or groups of muscles. The lesion is located in the anterior horn cells of the spinal cord, nerve roots, peripheral nerves, myoneural junctions, or muscles.

In the history, is there:
1. **Diffuse involvement?** Consider malabsorption syndrome, malnutrition, Simmonds' disease, Addison's disease, hyperthyroidism, cirrhosis, or metastatic neoplasm.
2. **Symmetric atrophy, but localized to proximal or distal muscle groups?** Consider muscular dystrophy or peripheral neuropathy.
3. **Asymmetric atrophy?** Consider amyotrophic lateral sclerosis, herniated disc, early spinal cord tumor, or entrapment neuropathies.
4. **Acute onset?** Consider poliomyelitis and Guillain-Barré syndrome.
5. **Pain in the involved extremity?** Consider a herniated disc.

On physical examination, is (are) there:
1. **Fasciculations?** Consider amyotrophic lateral sclerosis or nerve root involvement.
2. **Glove and stocking hypesthesia and hypalgesia?** Consider peripheral neuropathy.
3. **Dermatomal sensory loss?** Consider radiculopathy from a herniated disc or other space-occupying lesion of the spinal cord.
4. **A pelvic tilt?** Consider muscular dystrophy.
5. **A sensory level?** Consider a spinal cord tumor or syringomyelia.
6. **Cataracts?** Consider myotonic dystrophy.

Diagnostic Workup
1. Complete blood count (malabsorption syndrome)
2. Chemistry panel (cirrhosis, uremia)
3. Electromyography and nerve conduction velocity studies (amyotrophic lateral sclerosis)
4. Antinuclear antibody titer (dermatomyositis)
5. CT scan or MRI of the spine (space-occupying lesion of the spinal cord, herniated disc)
6. Muscle biopsy (muscular dystrophy)
7. Acetylcholine receptor antibody titer (myasthenia gravis)

NUCHAL RIGIDITY

Nuchal rigidity is the inability of the patient or the examiner to flex the patient's neck beyond the neutral position. The lesion is located in the meninges or cervical spine.

In the history, is there:
1. **Fever?** Consider bacterial or viral meningitis or encephalitis, although subarachnoid hemorrhage may also be associated with fever.
2. **Hypertension?** This suggests the presence of a ruptured cerebral aneurysm or intracerebral hemorrhage with extension into the subarachnoid space.
3. **Coma?** This would favor cerebral hemorrhage over meningitis, but both may cause coma.
4. **Trauma?** Consider fractured cervical vertebra or traumatic subarachnoid hemorrhage.

On physical examination, is (are) there:
1. **Focal neurologic signs?** Consider cerebral abscess, cerebral hemorrhage, or viral encephalitis.
2. **Subhyaloid hemorrhage?** Consider subarachnoid hemorrhage.
3. **Pneumonia or systemic infection?** Consider bacterial meningitis.
4. **Poor mobility of the cervical spine and radiculopathy?** Consider cervical arthritis or spondylosis.
5. **Tremor?** Consider Parkinson's disease.

Diagnostic Workup
1. Complete blood count, sedimentation rate (meningitis)
2. Blood cultures (meningitis)
3. CT scan (subarachnoid hemorrhage)
4. Spinal fluid examination (meningitis, subarachnoid hemorrhage)
5. Radiography of the cervical spine (cervical spine fracture)
6. Bone scan (cervical spine fracture)

NYSTAGMUS

Nystagmus is the rapid back and forth (lateral) or up and down (vertical) movement of the eyeballs. It is usually induced by glancing to the right or left or up and down. The neurologic lesion may be in the middle or inner ear, vestibular nerve, brainstem, or cerebellum. The rare ocular nystagmus is caused by visual disturbances such as partial blindness.

In the history, is (are) there:
1. **Earache?** Consider otitis media, mastoiditis, or petrositis.
2. **Headaches?** Consider a space-occupying lesion of the brain or brainstem.
3. **Vertigo or deafness?** Consider Meniere's disease, otitis media, ototoxicity, cholesteatoma, or acoustic neuroma.
4. **Drug use?** Consider phenytoin, muscle relaxants, barbiturates, or aminoglycosides.

On physical examination, is (are) there:
1. **Abnormalities on the ear examination?** Suspect a foreign body, otitis media, perforation, or cholesteatoma.
2. **Vertical nystagmus?** Suspect a space-occupying lesion of the cerebellum or brainstem.
3. **Other cranial nerve involvement or long tract signs?** Suspect a space-occupying lesion of the brainstem, basilar artery insufficiency or aneurysm, multiple sclerosis, or hereditary ataxia.
4. **Papilledema?** Consider a space-occupying lesion of the cerebellum or brainstem.

Diagnostic Workup
1. Audiogram, caloric tests, or electronystagmography (Meniere's disease, acoustic neuroma)
2. Radiography of the mastoid process and petrous bones (mastoiditis, petrositis)
3. CT scan or MRI of the brain (acoustic neuroma or other space-occupying lesion, multiple sclerosis)
4. Four-vessel cerebral angiography (vertebral-basilar aneurysm or insufficiency)
5. Spinal tap (neurosyphilis, multiple sclerosis)
6. Ear, nose, and throat consultation

OPISTHOTONUS

Opisthotonus is the arching or hyperextension of the neck and the entire spine. The lesion is usually in the meninges.

In the history, is there:
1. **Drug use?** Opisthotonus is an adverse reaction of phenothiazine and haloperidol. Parenteral drug use with dirty needles may induce tetanus and opisthotonus.
2. **Fever?** Consider bacterial meningitis.
3. **Wound infection?** A dirty wound may lead to tetanus, which is associated with opisthotonus.
4. **Episodic opisthotonus?** Consider epilepsy as a possibility.

On physical examination, is there:
1. **Subhyaloid hemorrhage?** Suspect subarachnoid hemorrhage.

Diagnostic Workup
1. Complete blood count (meningitis, tetanus)
2. Blood cultures (meningitis)
3. Urine drug screen (drug intoxication)
4. CT scan (subarachnoid hemorrhage)
5. Spinal tap (meningitis, subarachnoid hemorrhage)
6. EEG, awake and asleep (epilepsy)

PAPILLEDEMA

Papilledema is swelling or edema of the optic disc. The lesion is usually located in the optic nerve or is the result of an increase in intracranial pressure leading to congestion of the veins feeding the disc.

In the history, is (are) there:
1. **Hypertension?** Malignant hypertension is an occasional cause of papilledema.
2. **Scotoma?** Consider optic neuritis.
3. **Headaches without hypertension?** Suspect a space-occupying lesion of the brain.
4. **Trauma?** Suspect a subdural or epidural hematoma.
5. **A female patient with obesity?** Consider the possibility of pseudotumor cerebri.
6. **Shortness of breath?** Consider the possibility of a chronic respiratory disorder, such as emphysema.

On physical examination, is (are) there:
1. **A central scotoma on visual field examination?** Suspect optic neuritis.
2. **Signs of long tract or cranial nerve involvement?** Suspect a space-occupying lesion of the brain or multiple sclerosis.
3. **Plethora?** Consider polycythemia.
4. **Hypertension?** Consider malignant hypertension.

Diagnostic Workup
1. Visual field examination (optic neuritis)
2. CT scan or MRI of the brain (space-occupying lesion)
3. Spinal tap (multiple sclerosis, pseudotumor cerebri). Do not perform a spinal tap unless a CT scan or MRI has been done to rule out a space-occupying lesion.
4. Hypertensive workup (asymptomatic hypertension)

PTOSIS

Ptosis is drooping of the eyelid, either partially or completely. The lesion may be in the brainstem, oculomotor nerve, myoneural junction, or muscle. It may also be in the sympathetic pathways (Horner syndrome; see page 67).

In the history, is there:
1. **Intermittent ptosis?** Consider myasthenia gravis or migraine.
2. **Diabetes?** Consider diabetic neuropathy.
3. **Acute onset?** Suspect cerebral aneurysm, diabetic neuropathy, or stroke.
4. **Gradual onset?** Suspect neoplasm or degenerative disorder.
5. **Diplopia?** Suspect oculomotor nerve involvement.

On physical examination, is (are) there:
1. **Constricted pupil?** Consider Horner syndrome (see page 67).
2. **Dilated pupil?** Suspect an aneurysm of the circle of Willis.
3. **Papilledema?** Suspect a brain tumor.
4. **Bilateral ptosis with evidence of symmetric wasting and weakness of the muscles of the extremities?** Consider muscular dystrophy.
5. **Other cranial nerve involvement?** Suspect cavernous sinus thrombosis, tuberculous meningitis, syphilitic meningitis, or brainstem glioma.
6. **Hyperactive reflexes?** Consider syringobulbia, platybasia, brainstem tumor, vertebral basilar artery occlusion or insufficiency, or multiple sclerosis.
7. **Hypoactive reflexes?** This would suggest myotonic dystrophy.

Diagnostic Workup
1. Glucose tolerance test (diabetic neuropathy)
2. CT scan or MRI of the brain (aneurysm or brain tumor)
3. Cerebral angiography (cerebral aneurysm or stroke)
4. Response to intravenous thiamine (Wernicke's encephalopathy)
5. Tensilon test (myasthenia gravis)

RISUS SARDONICUS

Risus sardonicus is a fixed grin due to a spasm of the facial muscles.

In the history, is (are) there:
1. **Parenteral drug use or wound infection?** Consider tetanus.
2. **Symptoms of mental illness?** Consider the possibility of strychnine poisoning.
3. **Skin disease?** Consider scleroderma.

On physical examination, is (are) there:
1. **Multiple injection marks?** Consider tetanus.
2. **Nonpitting edema of the hands and feet?** Look for scleroderma.
3. **Raynaud's phenomenon?** Look for scleroderma.

Diagnostic Workup
1. Wound smear and cultures (tetanus)
2. Urine drug screen (narcotic addiction)
3. Complete blood count and sedimentation rate (infection, scleroderma)
4. Psychometric testing (hysteria, depression)
5. Psychometric consultation

ROMBERG'S SIGN

Romberg's sign is present when the patient is unable to maintain his or her balance while standing with the feet close together and the eyes closed. The lesion is usually located in the posterior columns, dorsal nerve roots, or peripheral nerves, but it may be located in the vestibular system. Involvement of the cerebellum and cerebellar tracts may produce unsteadiness in the Romberg position, but this unsteadiness does not increase appreciably when the patient closes his or her eyes.

In the history, is (are) there:
1. **Alcoholism?** Consider peripheral neuropathy secondary to alcohol.
2. **A familial disorder of the nervous system?** Consider Friedreich's ataxia or peroneal muscular atrophy.
3. **Vertigo?** Consider a vestibular disorder, such as Meniere's disease.
4. **Lightning-like pains in the extremities?** Suspect tabes dorsalis.
5. **Radicular pain?** Suspect a spinal cord tumor.

On physical examination, is (are) there:
1. **Pallor?** Consider pernicious anemia.
2. **Nystagmus?** Suspect a vestibular or cerebellar disorder.
3. **Argyll Robertson pupils?** Suspect tabes dorsalis.
4. **Glove and stocking hypesthesia and hypalgesia?** This would suggest a peripheral neuropathy.
5. **Pathologic reflexes?** Consider pernicious anemia, multiple sclerosis, or Friedreich's ataxia.
6. **Central scotoma?** Suspect multiple sclerosis.
7. **Papilledema?** Look for cerebellar tumor.

Diagnostic Workup
1. Complete blood count (pernicious anemia)
2. Venereal Disease Research Laboratory (VDRL) test (tabes dorsalis)
3. Serum vitamin B_{12} level (pernicious anemia)
4. Antinuclear antibody titer (peripheral neuropathy)
5. Nerve conduction velocity studies (peripheral neuropathy)
6. Somatosensory evoked potentials (multiple sclerosis)
7. MRI of the spine (neoplasm, multiple sclerosis, Friedreich's ataxia)
8. MRI of the brain (space-occupying lesion of the brain)
9. Spinal tap (neurosyphilis, multiple sclerosis)
10. Neuropathy workup (see Peripheral neuropathy in Appendix B)

SENSORY LOSS

Loss of sensation may present in a variety of ways. Sensory loss may be diffuse or focal; it may involve only one modality or all modalities. The lesion may be located in the peripheral nerves, sensory root, spinal cord, brainstem, or brain.

In the history, is there:
1. **Involvement of only one extremity?** Consider the possibility of radiculopathy, entrapment neuropathy, or sciatic or brachial plexus neuropathy.
2. **Pain associated with the sensory loss?** Suspect radiculopathy or tabes dorsalis.
3. **Headache?** Consider the possibility of a space-occupying lesion of the brain.
4. **Acute onset?** Suspect cerebrovascular disease, infection, trauma, or multiple sclerosis.
5. **Gradual onset?** This suggests a neoplasm or degenerative disorder.
6. **Episodic occurrence?** This suggests demyelination disease or transient ischemic attack.

On physical examination, is (are) there:
1. **Involvement of the face only?** Suspect acoustic neuroma or petrositis.
2. **Involvement of the face on one side and extremities on the other?** Suspect a posterior inferior cerebellar artery occlusion or basilar artery insufficiency.
3. **Involvement of one-half of the body?** Suspect a thalamic syndrome.
4. **Dermatomal loss of sensation?** Suspect a herniated disc, neoplasm of the spinal cord, or other causes of radiculopathy.
5. **A sensory level?** Suspect a space-occupying lesion of the spinal cord.
6. **Loss of vibratory and position sense on one side, and pain and temperature sense on the other?** Consider a spinal cord tumor with Brown-Séquard syndrome.
7. **Sacral sparing?** Suspect an intramedullary tumor or syringomyelia.
8. **Symmetric loss of vibratory and position sense only?** Suspect pernicious anemia, Friedreich's ataxia, tabes dorsalis, multiple sclerosis, or parasagittal neoplasm.
9. **Glove and stocking hypesthesia and hypalgesia?** Suspect a peripheral neuropathy.

Diagnostic Workup
1. Complete blood count (pernicious anemia)
2. Serum vitamin B_{12} level (pernicious anemia)
3. Venereal Disease Research Laboratory (VDRL) test (neurosyphilis)
4. Antinuclear antibody titer (peripheral neuropathy)
5. Neuropathy workup (see Appendix B)
6. MRI of the spine (space-occupying lesion, herniated disc, multiple sclerosis, degenerative disorder)
7. MRI of the brain (space-occupying lesion, cerebrovascular disease, multiple sclerosis, degenerative disorder)
8. Spinal tap (neurosyphilis, multiple sclerosis)
9. Nerve conduction velocity studies (entrapment neuropathies, peripheral neuropathy, radiculopathy)
10. Somatosensory evoked potentials (multiple sclerosis)

SPASTICITY

Spasticity is continuous tension of the muscles of the extremities or face, causing joint stiffness and disturbance of motion. The lesion may be located in the pyramidal tracts from the spinal cord to the brain, or in the basal ganglia.

In the history, is there:
1. **Birth trauma or anoxia?** This suggests cerebral palsy.
2. **Gradual onset?** This suggests a neoplasm or degenerative disorder. It may also indicate stiff-man syndrome.
3. **Acute onset?** This suggests a vascular or inflammatory disorder.
4. **Episodic occurrence?** Suspect epilepsy or transient ischemic attack.

On physical examination, is there:
1. **Diffuse involvement, with tremor and cogwheel rigidity?** Suspect Parkinson's disease or other extrapyramidal disorder.
2. **Hemiplegia?** Suspect a vascular, neoplastic, or traumatic lesion of the brain or brainstem.
3. **Paraplegia or quadriplegia, without cranial nerve involvement?** Suspect a space-occupying lesion of the spinal cord, anterior spinal artery occlusion, degenerative disorder, trauma, or multiple sclerosis. Also consider stiff-man syndrome.
4. **Paraplegia or quadriplegia, with cranial nerve involvement?** Suspect brainstem neoplasm, vascular disease, degenerative disorder, or multiple sclerosis.

Diagnostic Workup
1. Serum copper and ceruloplasmin levels (Wilson's disease)
2. Heavy metal screen (manganese toxicity)
3. MRI of the spinal cord (space-occupying lesion, multiple sclerosis)
4. MRI of the brain (space-occupying lesion of the brain, multiple sclerosis, stroke)
5. Four-vessel angiography (cerebrovascular disease)

TREMOR

Tremors are rhythmic oscillations of the fingers, hands, or other parts of the body. A tremor may occur while the patient is at rest or may occur on intention. In a tremor at rest, the lesion is usually located in the basal ganglia, whereas intention tremor is usually caused by a cerebellar lesion.

In the history, is (are) there:
1. **Nicotine, caffeine, or alcohol use?** Nicotine and caffeine produce a fine tremor, mainly on intention. Alcohol withdrawal (delirium tremens) is commonly associated with tremor.
2. **Drug use or abuse?** Prescription drugs such as barbiturates, phenytoin, phenothiazine, and lithium may cause tremor. Amphetamines, cocaine, and phencyclidine (PCP) are just a few of the illegal drugs that may cause tremor.
3. **Occupational exposure to heavy metals?** Manganese toxicity produces a parkinsonian syndrome, and lead, mercury, and other heavy metals may produce a fine tremor.
4. **Other family members affected?** Essential tremor and many cerebellar disorders are familial.
5. **Insulin-dependent diabetes?** Look for hypoglycemia.

On physical examination, is (are) there:
1. **An enlarged thyroid?** Consider hyperthyroidism.
2. **Rigidity, short-stepped gait, or monotonous speech?** This would suggest Parkinson's disease.
3. **Kayser-Fleischer ring or wing-flapping tremor of the arms?** Consider the possibility of Wilson's disease.
4. **Tremor on one side of the body only?** Consider the possibility of a thalamic syndrome or a contralateral frontal lobe tumor, abscess, or trauma.
5. **Ataxia and/or nystagmus?** Look for a cerebellar tumor, multiple sclerosis, hereditary cerebellar ataxia, or Wernicke's encephalopathy.

Diagnostic Workup
1. Thyroid profile (thyrotoxicosis)
2. Blood alcohol level (alcoholism)
3. Urine drug screen (drug intoxication)
4. Serum copper and ceruloplasmin levels (Wilson's disease)
5. Urine porphobilinogen level (porphyria)
6. Venereal Disease Research Laboratory (VDRL) test (general paresis)
7. Response to intravenous thiamine (Wernicke's encephalopathy)
8. Chemistry panel (hypoglycemia, uremia, liver failure)
9. CT scan or MRI of the brain (space-occupying lesion, multiple sclerosis)
10. Spinal tap (neurosyphilis, multiple sclerosis)

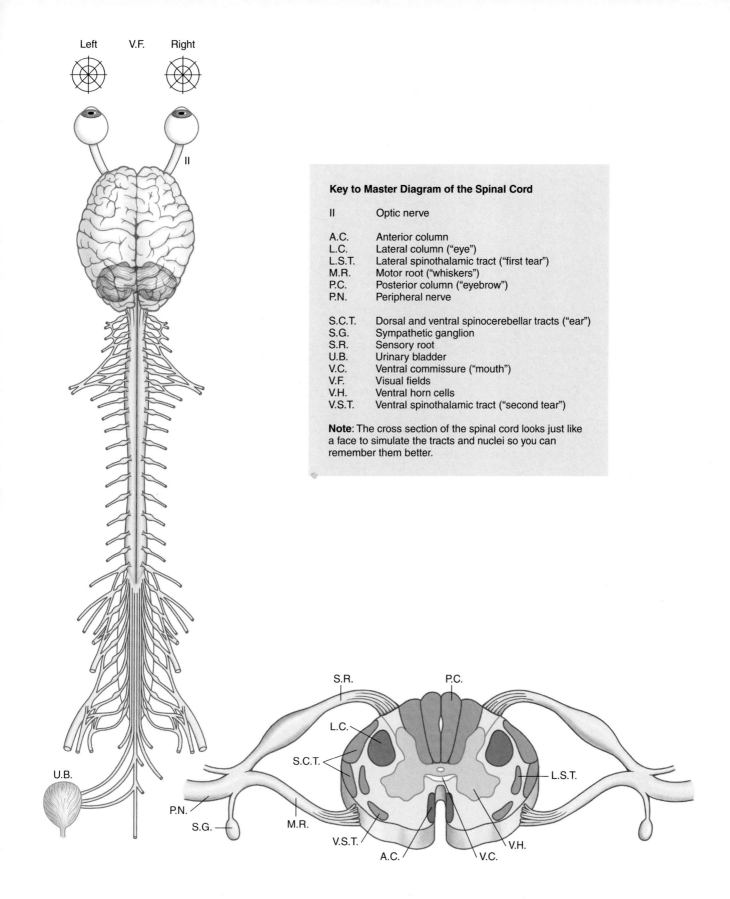

Left   V.F.   Right

II

Key to Master Diagram of the Spinal Cord

II   Optic nerve

A.C.   Anterior column
L.C.   Lateral column ("eye")
L.S.T.   Lateral spinothalamic tract ("first tear")
M.R.   Motor root ("whiskers")
P.C.   Posterior column ("eyebrow")
P.N.   Peripheral nerve

S.C.T.   Dorsal and ventral spinocerebellar tracts ("ear")
S.G.   Sympathetic ganglion
S.R.   Sensory root
U.B.   Urinary bladder
V.C.   Ventral commissure ("mouth")
V.F.   Visual fields
V.H.   Ventral horn cells
V.S.T.   Ventral spinothalamic tract ("second tear")

Note: The cross section of the spinal cord looks just like a face to simulate the tracts and nuclei so you can remember them better.

S.R.   P.C.
L.C.
S.C.T.
L.S.T.
U.B.
P.N.
S.G.   M.R.
V.S.T.   V.H.
A.C.   V.C.

PART THREE: Diseases of the Spinal Cord, Peripheral Nerves, and Muscles

Diseases of the Spinal Cord, Peripheral Nerves, and Muscles

ACUTE IDIOPATHIC POLYNEUROPATHY
(Guillain-Barré Syndrome)

Left   Right

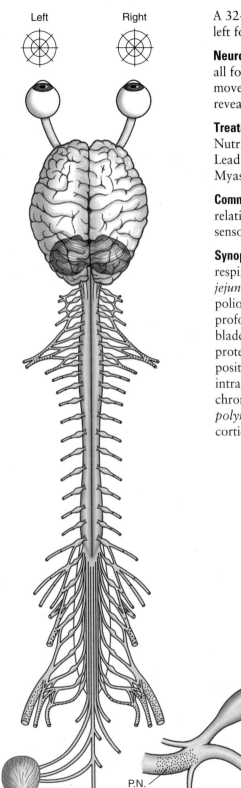

A 32-year-old white man complained of numbness and tingling in his right hand and left foot. A day later he developed weakness in all four extremities.

Neurologic examination revealed bilateral facial palsy, weakness and hyporeflexia of all four extremities, diminished sensation to touch and pain, and total loss of movement in the left foot and toes and in the right thumb. Spinal fluid examination revealed a total protein of 410 mg/dL but no cells.

Treatable Diseases to Be Ruled Out
Nutritional neuropathy
Lead neuropathy
Myasthenia gravis

Comment: The diffuse, patchy demyelination of the peripheral nerves is illustrated in a relatively symmetric fashion and is responsible for the weakness, areflexia, and sensory loss.

Synopsis: Acute idiopathic polyneuropathy develops most commonly after an upper respiratory infection, surgical procedure, vaccination, or a preceding *Campylobacter jejuni* infection, so it is presumed to be autoimmune in nature. In contrast to poliomyelitis, there are usually sensory deficits and the attack on the brainstem is less profound, although there may be dysarthria and dysphagia. Both diseases affect bladder function and respiration. Diagnosis is established by a high spinal fluid protein with a disproportionately low cell count. Nerve conduction studies are positive for peripheral neuropathy. Treatment is supportive, but plasmapheresis and intravenous immunoglobulin may be beneficial (see Appendix C for details). A chronic form of this disorder, called *chronic inflammatory demyelinating polyneuropathy*, exists but is rare. Patients with chronic disease respond to corticosteroids as well as immunoglobulin and plasmapheresis.

S.R.

P.N.

M.R.

Figure 1. Spinal Cord: Acute Idiopathic Polyneuropathy

AMYOTROPHIC LATERAL SCLEROSIS

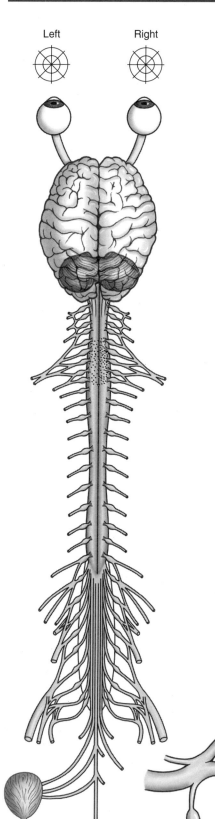

A 34-year-old white man complained of difficulty buttoning his clothes and holding onto things for the past 3 months.

Neurologic examination disclosed weakness of flexion, extension, adduction, and abduction of the fingers of both the patient's hands, but the weakness was more marked in his right hand. Atrophy and fasciculations were noted in the hypothenar and interossei muscles bilaterally, but these also were more marked in his right hand. Patellar and Achilles reflexes were hyperactive.

Treatable Diseases to Be Ruled Out
Spinal cord tumor
Herniated disc
Cervical spondylosis
Tuberculosis of the spine
Nutritional neuropathy
Neurosyphilis

Comment: Note the involvement of the anterior horn cells, leading to weakness, atrophy, and fasciculations, and of the pyramidal tracts, causing weakness and hyperactive reflexes in the lower extremities. Amyotrophic lateral sclerosis usually spares the extraocular muscles, sensory nerves, sphincters.

Synopsis: Amyotrophic lateral sclerosis is a devastating degenerative disease of the motor horn cells and pyramidal tracts in the brainstem or spinal cord. The etiology is unknown, except in the small number of familial cases. Cases in which the patient presents with purely lower motor neuron disease are labeled *progressive muscular atrophy*, whereas those in which the patient presents with purely upper motor neuron disease are labeled *primary lateral sclerosis*. Whether these two types of cases are distinct entities is debatable. Amyotrophic lateral sclerosis is slowly progressive, with death from respiratory failure in 3 to 4 years in most cases. There is no known cure, but riluzole (100 mg daily) may slow the progression of the disease and reduce mortality. Otherwise, treatment is supportive (see Appendix C). Diagnosis is by exclusion of other disorders with nerve conduction velocity studies, electromyography, and MRI of the cervical spine.

Figure 2. Spinal Cord: Amyotrophic Lateral Sclerosis

ANTERIOR SPINAL ARTERY OCCLUSION

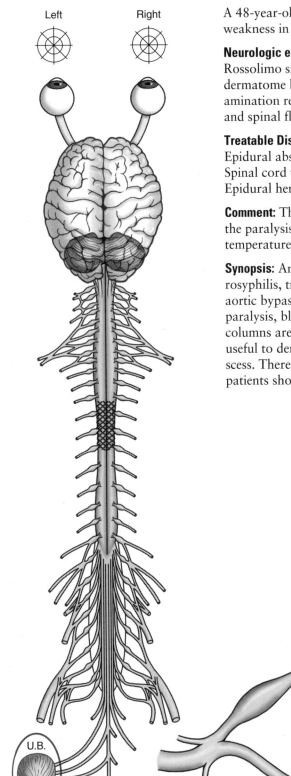

A 48-year-old black woman with a known history of lues had a sudden onset of weakness in her lower extremities and bladder retention.

Neurologic examination revealed flaccid paralysis of both lower extremities, bilateral Rossolimo signs, and loss of sensation to pain and temperature below the T5 dermatome bilaterally. Vibratory and position senses were preserved. Laboratory examination revealed positive fluorescent treponemal antibody absorption in the blood and spinal fluid.

Treatable Diseases to Be Ruled Out
Epidural abscess
Spinal cord tumor
Epidural hematoma

Comment: The illustration shows involvement of the pyramidal tracts (accounting for the paralysis) and the lateral spinothalamic tracts (accounting for the loss of pain and temperature).

Synopsis: Anterior spinal artery occlusion is rare but may be associated with neurosyphilis, trauma, dissecting aneurysm of the aorta, embolism, collagen disease, or aortic bypass surgery. This case illustrates the typical clinical presentation with flaccid paralysis, bladder dysfunction, and dissociative sensory loss because the posterior columns are supplied by the posterior spinal arteries. An MRI of the spinal cord is useful to demonstrate the lesion and rule out treatable disorders such as epidural abscess. There is no specific treatment. The prognosis for full recovery is poor, but many patients show considerable improvement over several months.

Figure 3. Spinal Cord: Anterior Spinal Artery Occlusion

CARPAL TUNNEL SYNDROME

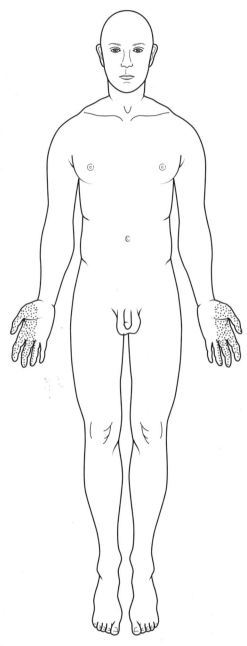

Figure 1. Spinal Cord: Carpal Tunnel Syndrome

A 23-year-old computer operator complained of numbness and tingling in both hands, with both symptoms being worse in the right hand.

Neurologic examination revealed hypesthesia and hypalgesia in both hands on the volar surfaces of the thumbs, index fingers, middle fingers, and medial half of the ring fingers. The right thenar eminence was atrophied. Nerve conduction velocity studies confirmed the diagnosis.

Treatable Diseases to Be Ruled Out
Spinal cord tumor
Herniated cervical disc
Thoracic outlet syndrome
Ulnar neuropathy

Comment: The illustration shows the loss of sensation to touch and pain in the median nerve distribution bilaterally.

Synopsis: Carpal tunnel syndrome is usually an occupation-related condition resulting from compression of the median nerve as it passes through the carpal tunnel in the wrist. It may also result from rheumatoid arthritis, acromegaly, pregnancy, amyloidosis, myxedema, or multiple myeloma. Any form of arthritis or collagen disease may be responsible. Diagnosis is confirmed by the clinical picture and nerve conduction velocity studies. Carpal tunnel syndrome may be treated conservatively with high-dose pyridoxine (vitamin B_6) therapy or corticosteroid injection into the tunnel (see Appendix C). Ultimately, surgical decompression may be necessary.

CERVICAL SPONDYLOSIS

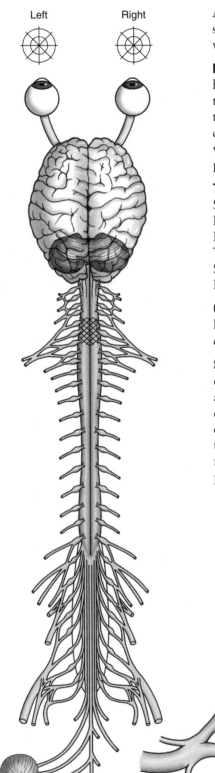

Left   Right

A 47-year-old Polish laborer experienced intermittent, severe pain in his neck and shoulders for the past year. For the past 3 months, he dragged his feet when he walked and was unsteady on his feet, especially in the dark.

Neurologic examination disclosed mild atrophy and weakness of the left shoulder and hand muscles. There were hyperactive patellar and Achilles reflexes bilaterally. Sensation to touch and pain was diminished in the thumb and index fingers bilaterally, and there was loss of vibratory and position senses below the knees. A radiograph of the cervical spine showed narrowing of the disc spaces at C5-C6 and C6-C7 associated with prominent osteoarthritic spurring. An MRI demonstrated root and cord compression at the C5-C6 interspace. The cervical canal measured 12 mm in diameter.

Treatable Diseases to Be Ruled Out
Spinal cord tumor
Herniated disc
Epidural abscess
Tuberculosis of the spine
Syphilitic meningomyelitis
Epidural or subdural hematoma

Comment: The illustration shows involvement of the posterior column (causing the loss of vibratory and position senses), lateral columns (causing weakness and increased reflexes in the lower extremities), and nerve roots at C5 and C6.

Synopsis: Cervical spondylosis results from degeneration of the cervical discs with secondary osteophytic reaction, leading to encroachment of the intervertebral foramina and spinal canal. Patients with a congenitally narrow spinal canal (12 mm or less in diameter) are particularly vulnerable. The diagnosis is established by plain films of the cervical spine and an MRI. It is rarely necessary to do combined CT and myelography to confirm the diagnosis. Conservative treatment with traction and physiotherapy may be adequate if there is only root involvement, but when there is spinal cord compression, a laminectomy or anterior body fusion is necessary.

S.R.   P.C.

L.C.

M.R.

Figure 2. Spinal Cord: Cervical Spondylosis

COMPRESSION FRACTURE OF THE SPINE

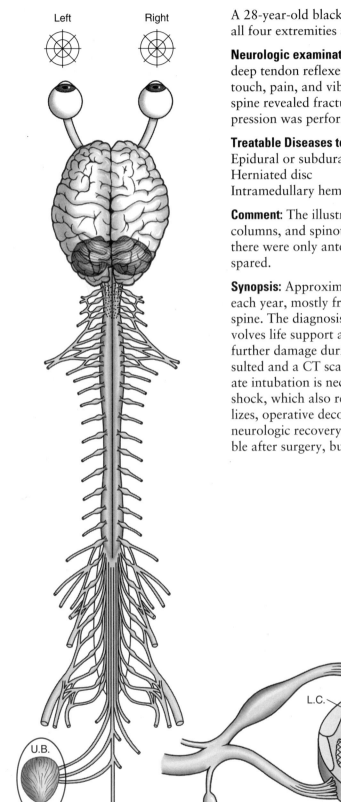

Left   Right

U.B.

A 28-year-old black man was brought to the emergency department unable to move all four extremities after an automobile accident.

Neurologic examination revealed flaccid paralysis of all four extremities and loss of all deep tendon reflexes. The bladder was percussed above the umbilicus. Sensation to touch, pain, and vibration was lost below the neck. A roentgenogram of the cervical spine revealed fractures of the sixth and seventh cervical vertebrae. Operative decompression was performed.

Treatable Diseases to Be Ruled Out
Epidural or subdural hematoma
Herniated disc
Intramedullary hematoma

Comment: The illustration shows the involvement of the pyramidal tracts, posterior columns, and spinothalamic tracts producing the clinical picture described above. If there were only anterior spinal artery occlusion, the posterior columns would be spared.

Synopsis: Approximately 10,000 cases of spinal cord injury occur in the United States each year, mostly from auto accidents. About half of these injuries affect the cervical spine. The diagnosis is established by a CT scan or MRI. Immediate treatment involves life support and carefully placing a hard cervical collar on the neck to prevent further damage during transport. Upon arrival at the hospital, a neurosurgeon is consulted and a CT scan or MRI is done. If diaphragmatic paralysis is suspected, immediate intubation is necessary along with mechanical ventilation. The patient may be in shock, which also requires immediate treatment. Once the patient's condition stabilizes, operative decompression must be done if he or she is to have any chance for neurologic recovery. A program of physiotherapy should be started as soon as possible after surgery, but the prognosis for good neurologic recovery is guarded.

P.C.

L.C.

L.S.T.

Figure 3. Spinal Cord: Compression Fracture of the Spine

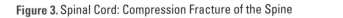

DIABETIC NEUROPATHY

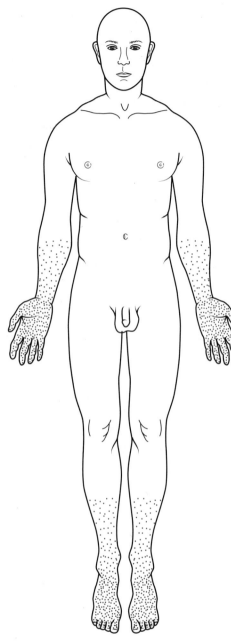

Figure 1. Spinal Cord: Diabetic Neuropathy

A 58-year-old man with diabetes complained of weakness, numbness, and tingling in all four extremities for several months.

Neurologic examination revealed weakness and atrophy of the small hand muscles bilaterally; loss of sensation to touch, pain, and vibration distally in all four extremities; and a steppage gait. Nerve conduction velocity studies confirmed the diagnosis.

Treatable Diseases to Be Ruled Out
Nutritional neuropathy
Lead neuropathy
Collagen disease
Pernicious anemia
Neurosyphilis

Comment: The illustration demonstrates the distal loss of sensation to pain, touch, and vibration in a symmetric distribution in all four extremities.

Synopsis: Diabetes is the most common cause of peripheral neuropathy. Diabetic neuropathy may present as a symmetric polyneuropathy or a mononeuropathy such as Bell's palsy or oculomotor palsy. The neuropathy seems to be associated with poor control of hyperglycemia. The mononeuropathy is associated with focal abnormalities of the vasa nervorum or with angiopathic injury. Diagnosis is usually not difficult in the setting of long-standing insulin-dependent diabetes. Nerve conduction velocity studies are usually necessary, but nerve biopsy is rarely required. Treatment includes good control of hyperglycemia, proper nutrition, and a multiple vitamin B supplement. Bothersome dysesthesia and lightning-like pains may be treated with antiepileptic drugs and tricyclic antidepressants.

EPIDURAL ABSCESS

Left   Right

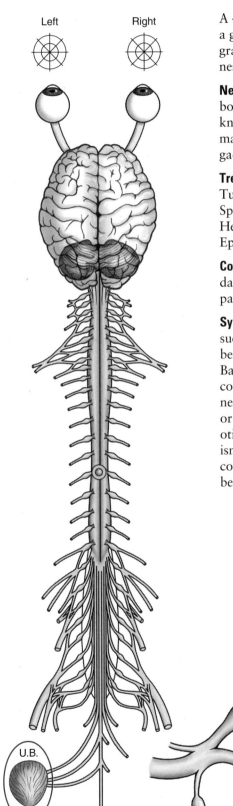

A 48-year-old woman with diabetes developed a rather sudden, severe backache and a girdle-like pain around her chest that worsened when she sneezed. A chest radiograph and ECG were normal. A few days later, she developed fever, chills, and weakness in both legs.

Neurologic examination revealed weakness, hyperactive reflexes, and Babinski signs in both lower extremities. Vibratory and position senses were diminished below the knee, and there was a sensory level at T8 bilaterally. The urine sample contained many gram-positive cocci, indicating a possible source for the infection. An MRI with gadolinium enhancement demonstrated the lesion.

Treatable Diseases to Be Ruled Out
Tuberculoma
Spinal cord tumor
Herniated disc
Epidural hematoma

Comment: The illustration shows the abscess, with cord compression causing pyramidal tract, posterior column, and lateral spinothalamic tract dysfunction, leading to the patient's symptoms and signs.

Synopsis: Epidural abscess is usually secondary to an infection elsewhere in the body, such as cellulitis, pyelonephritis (as in this case), or osteomyelitis. The condition may be an extension of tuberculosis of the spine, in which case the onset is more gradual. Back trauma, surgery, or lumbar puncture may be the cause. The diagnosis is best confirmed by MRI, but if this test is not available, a CT scan or myelography may be necessary. Plain films and a bone scan will help diagnose an associated osteomyelitis or tuberculosis of the spine. Treatment is usually surgical decompression and antibiotics for several weeks based on the results of culture of the lesion. Because the organism most likely involved is *Staphylococcus aureus* or *Streptococcus*, nafcillin or vancomycin is begun while the clinician awaits the results of the culture. Dosages should be in the range required for meningitis (see Appendix C).

Figure 1. Spinal Cord: Epidural Abscess

FIBROMYALGIA

A 42-year-old white woman complained of pain in almost all her joints, sensitivity to cold, throbbing pain in her shoulders, stiffness in her feet and ankles, and a prickly feeling in her legs since a total hysterectomy 6 months ago.

Neurologic examination, joint examination, and general physical examination were normal. Laboratory examination failed to confirm joint disease or other pathology. Further history indicated she was on anti-inflammatory drugs, narcotics, and tricyclic antidepressants. There was a long history of treatment for mild depression.

Comment: This patient undoubtedly would be diagnosed with fibromyalgia (e.g., myofasciitis) by many physicians, but how can we put this kind of label on someone when there is no objective physical or laboratory evidence of disease? It is more reasonable to classify this condition as a low pain threshold. There are at least four possible explanations for the low pain threshold in this case: a long history of depression, narcotic use, the combination of antidepressants with other drugs, and surgically induced menopause. A battery of psychometric tests is indicated along with psychiatric consultation. Just as important is the elimination of all drugs, especially narcotics, for a considerable period of time (it takes months to eliminate some of these drugs from the system).

FRIEDREICH'S ATAXIA

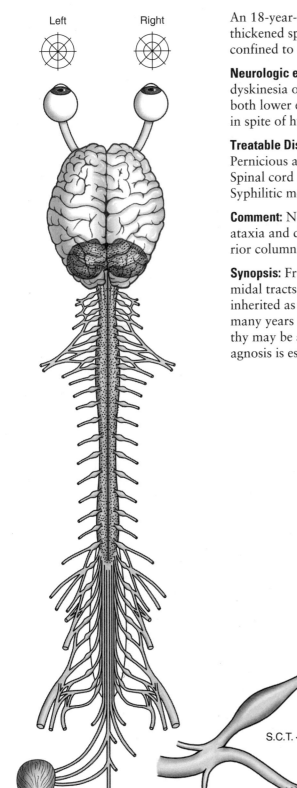

An 18-year-old white man was brought for examination because of unsteady gait, thickened speech, and clumsiness of his hands for the past year. His uncle had been confined to a wheelchair at age 26.

Neurologic examination revealed horizontal nystagmus; slurred, monotonous speech; dyskinesia on rapid alternation testing; impairment of vibratory and position senses in both lower extremities; and a lurching, ataxic gait. There were bilateral Babinski signs in spite of hypoactive reflexes. Of particular note were hammer toes and pes cavus.

Treatable Diseases to Be Ruled Out
Pernicious anemia
Spinal cord tumor
Syphilitic meningomyelitis

Comment: Note the involvement of the spinocerebellar tracts, accounting for the ataxia and dyskinesia; the lateral column, causing the Babinski signs; and the posterior columns, causing the loss of vibratory and position senses.

Synopsis: Friedreich's ataxia is a slowly progressive, degenerative disease of the pyramidal tracts, dorsal root ganglia, posterior columns, and spinocerebellar tracts. It is inherited as an autosomal recessive trait. It usually begins in childhood and takes many years to develop. Treatment is supportive, as there is no cure. A cardiomyopathy may be associated with this disorder and is frequently the cause of death. The diagnosis is established by genetic testing.

Figure 1. Spinal Cord: Friedreich's Ataxia

HERNIATED DISC (LUMBAR)

Left   Right

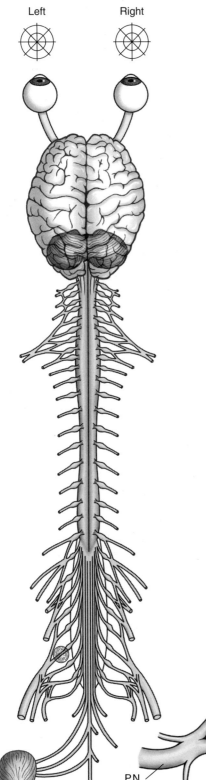

A 33-year-old black laborer developed severe lancinating pain radiating down the posterior aspect of his left thigh while he was lifting a heavy steel beam.

Neurologic examination disclosed slight lumbar scoliosis to the right, weakness of dorsiflexion and plantar flexion of the left fourth and fifth toes, absent left Achilles reflex, hypalgesia of the lateral aspect of the left lower leg and foot, and a positive Lasègue sign. Routine laboratory studies and radiographs of the lumbar spine were negative, but MRI of the lumbar spine showed a large herniated disc at the L5-S1 interspace, confirming the diagnosis.

Treatable Diseases to Be Ruled Out
Epidural abscess
Pelvic tumor
Cauda equina tumor
Multiple myeloma
Metastatic carcinoma
Tuberculosis of the spinal column

Comment: Note that in the illustration, the disc is compressing the ventral root, causing weakness in dorsiflexion of the left fourth and fifth toes, and the dorsal root, causing hypalgesia of the left lower leg and foot.

Synopsis: Herniated lumbar discs are a common work-related injury and are almost always related to trauma, especially from heavy lifting. The symptoms of low back and leg pain are usually acute in onset and associated with paresthesia and sensory loss in the involved nerve roots, as well as weakness, loss of reflexes, and atrophy as the disease progresses. The most common roots affected are L4, L5, and S1. Ninety percent of patients respond to conservative treatment within 4 to 6 weeks, so an aggressive surgical approach is not called for unless a cauda equina syndrome with bladder involvement is identified. In the diagnostic workup, routine laboratory tests are negative but need to be done in persistent cases and in the elderly, to rule out multiple myeloma (serum protein electrophoresis) and prostatic carcinoma (prostate-specific antigen). The same applies to radiography of the lumbar spine. The diagnostic procedure of choice is MRI of the lumbar spine, but it should only be undertaken if surgery is contemplated. CT scans and lumbar myelography are rarely indicated today. Treatment consists of conservative measures including physiotherapy, muscle relaxants, anti-inflammatory agents, and epidural steroids. If these measures fail to alleviate the pain in 6 to 8 weeks or if there is definite weakness or atrophy of the involved extremity, surgery is indicated. Microsurgical diskectomy, percutaneous diskectomy, and hemilaminectomy all have their advocates. The procedure of choice should be based on the experience of the neurosurgeon.

S.R.

P.N.

M.R.

Figure 1. Spinal Cord: Herniated Disc (Lumbar)

HERNIATED DISC (CERVICAL)

Left   Right

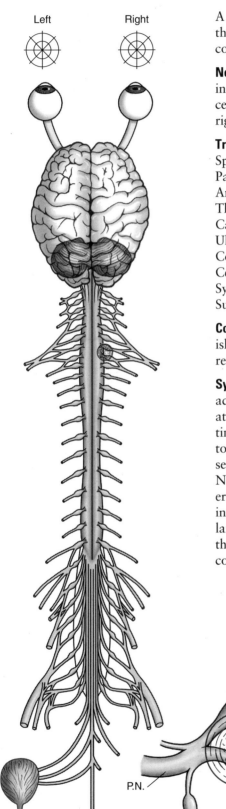

A 63-year-old black man complained of severe lancinating pain that radiated down the medial aspect of his right arm and forearm. Hyperextension of the cervical spine, coughing, and sneezing increased the pain, but exercise did not.

Neurologic examination revealed diminished sensation to touch and pain in the right index and middle fingers as well as a diminished right triceps reflex. An MRI of the cervical spine demonstrated a herniated disc at the C6-C7 interspace impinging on the right C7 nerve root.

Treatable Diseases to Be Ruled Out
Spinal cord tumor
Pancoast's tumor
Angina pectoris
Thoracic outlet syndrome
Carpal tunnel syndrome
Ulnar entrapment
Compression fracture
Cervical spondylosis
Sympathetic dystrophy
Subdeltoid bursitis

Comment: The illustration shows the disc compressing the sensory root, causing diminished sensation to touch and pain, and the motor root, causing loss of the triceps reflex.

Synopsis: Cervical disc herniation, like lumbar disc herniation, is usually traumatic. In addition to heavy lifting, hyperextension injuries may be the etiology. Cervical herniated discs are more likely to develop at a later age. Diagnostic workup includes routine laboratory studies, and radiography of the cervical spine is indicated at the onset to rule out osteoarthritis and metastatic carcinoma. When the pain persists after conservative treatment, MRI may be necessary, especially if surgery is contemplated. Nerve conduction velocity studies and electromyography are useful to rule out peripheral neuropathy, brachial plexus neuropathy, and entrapment syndromes. Treatment involves cervical traction and other physiotherapeutic measures along with muscle relaxants and anti-inflammatory drugs (see Appendix C). Surgery is indicated only if these measures have been unsuccessful or if definite atrophy or weakness occurs. Decompressive laminectomy, often with anterior body fusion, is the procedure of choice.

S.R.

P.N.

M.R.

Figure 2. Spinal Cord: Herniated Disc (Cervical)

HERPES ZOSTER

Left   Right

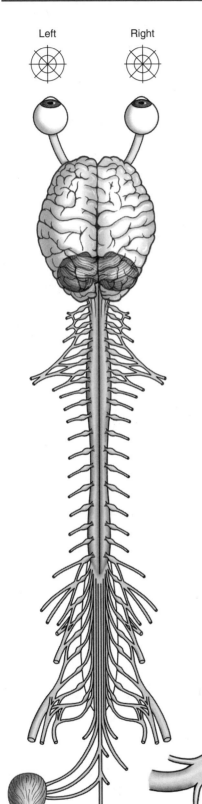

A 64-year-old white woman complained of severe pain in her left flank.

Neurologic examination revealed hyperesthesia in the distribution of the left twelfth thoracic nerve. Four days later, the patient developed a bullous eruption in the same distribution. Laboratory and roentgenographic examinations were normal.

Treatable Diseases to Be Ruled Out
Renal calculi
Pyelonephritis
Spinal cord tumor
Tuberculosis of the spine
Tabes dorsalis
Herniated disc

Comment: Note the involvement of the dorsal root ganglion, causing the severe pain and sensitivity to touch.

Synopsis: Herpes zoster is an inflammatory disease caused by the varicella virus, but it rarely affects children. It usually involves only the dorsal root ganglion, but in a few cases, it may spread into the spinal cord, brainstem, and brain. Patients with altered immunity due to Hodgkin's disease, HIV infection, or malignancy are particularly at risk. When the trigeminal nerve is involved, corneal ulceration may occur and must be treated as an emergency. Diagnosis is made by the clinical picture and exclusion of the other disorders listed above. Lumbar puncture may show lymphocytosis in many cases, especially if there is encephalitis. Treatment is symptomatic, as most cases are self-limited. A course of corticosteroids may be necessary to relieve pain (see Appendix C); acyclovir (800 mg every 4 hours) may be given to abort an attack. Postherpetic neuralgia is a complication, especially in the elderly, and may be treated with antiepileptic drugs (see Appendix C).

S.R.

Figure 3. Spinal Cord: Herpes Zoster

INFANTILE SPINAL MUSCULAR ATROPHY
(Werdnig-Hoffmann Disease)

Left   Right

A young mother complained that her 3-month-old daughter had difficulty swallowing and sucking and did not seem to be developing normally.

Neurologic examination revealed generalized flaccidity and weakness, loss of deep tendon reflexes, and atrophy and fasciculations of all four extremities. Electromyography revealed a diffuse neuropathic pattern. Genetic testing established the diagnosis.

Treatable Diseases to Be Ruled Out
Infectious polyneuritis
Lead neuropathy

Comment: Note that the illustration shows only anterior horn cell involvement, which leads to weakness, atrophy, and fasciculations, in contrast to amyotrophic lateral sclerosis, which is associated with pyramidal tract involvement.

Synopsis: Infantile spinal muscular atrophy is a hereditary progressive motor neuron disease that develops either in utero or in the first 3 months of life and progresses to respiratory failure and death during infancy. It is an autosomal recessive form of inheritance. Another form of this disease begins in childhood and has been labeled *Kugelberg-Welander syndrome*. Both forms are diagnosed by genetic testing, although electromyography and muscle biopsy are helpful in differentiating the disease from other disorders. There is no specific treatment available for Werdnig-Hoffmann disease or Kugelberg-Welander syndrome.

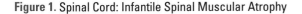

V.H.

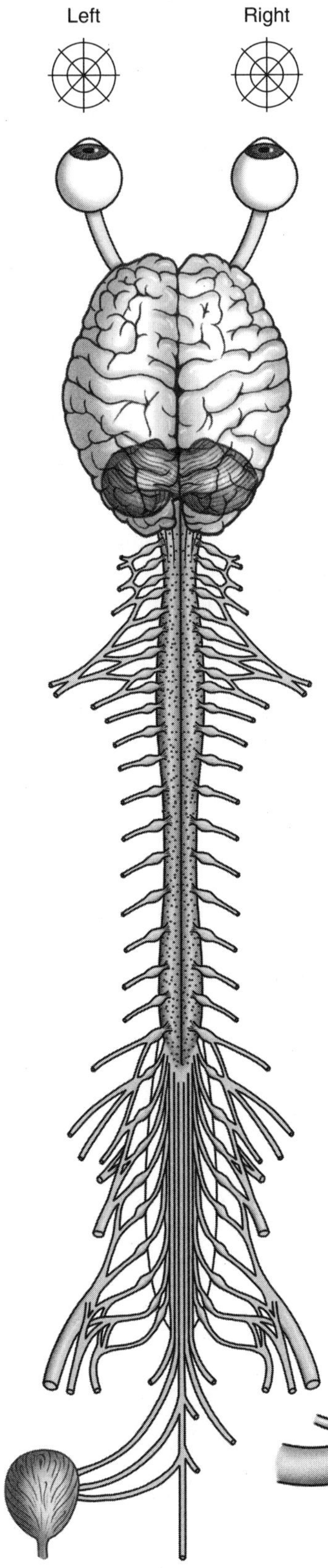

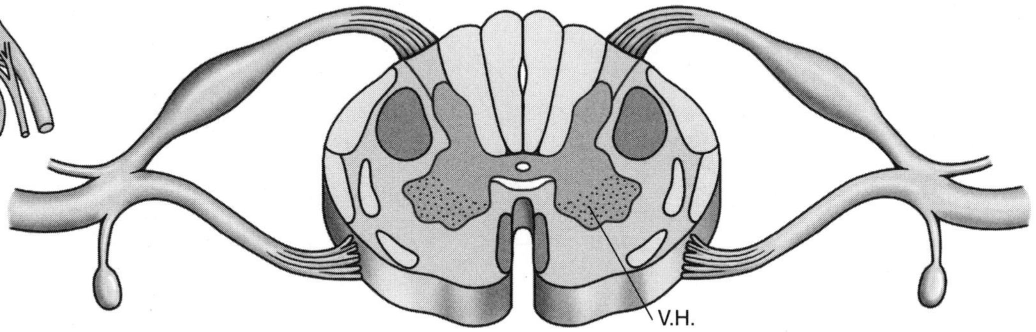

Figure 1. Spinal Cord: Infantile Spinal Muscular Atrophy

LEAD NEUROPATHY

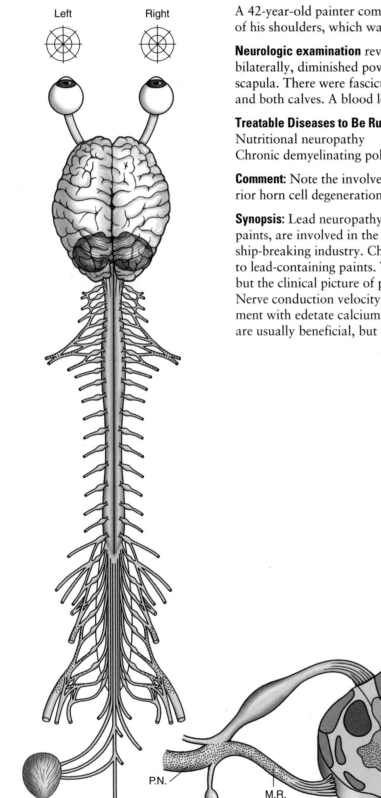

A 42-year-old painter complained of an inability to raise his right arm above the level of his shoulders, which was affecting his ability to do his job.

Neurologic examination revealed mild weakness of extension of the hands and fingers bilaterally, diminished power of dorsiflexion of the left foot, and winging of the right scapula. There were fasciculations and moderate atrophy in the right shoulder girdle and both calves. A blood lead level test confirmed the diagnosis.

Treatable Diseases to Be Ruled Out
Nutritional neuropathy
Chronic demyelinating polyneuropathy

Comment: Note the involvement of the peripheral nerves with secondary axonal anterior horn cell degeneration.

Synopsis: Lead neuropathy occurs primarily in individuals who use lead-containing paints, are involved in the repair or manufacture of storage batteries, or work in the ship-breaking industry. Children may develop a lead encephalopathy from exposure to lead-containing paints. The diagnosis is made by determining the blood lead level, but the clinical picture of primarily asymmetric motor nerve involvement is helpful. Nerve conduction velocity studies are also useful in cases that are confusing. Treatment with edetate calcium disodium (EDTA) and oral penicillamine (see Appendix C) are usually beneficial, but the morbidity and mortality rates are still unacceptable.

Figure 1. Spinal Cord: Lead Neuropathy

MISCELLANEOUS MONONEUROPATHY

Ulnar neuropathy: Ulnar neuropathy occurs when the ulnar nerve is trapped within the cubital tunnel at the elbow or is damaged from repeated external pressure. A fracture of the medial epicondyle or a valgus deformity may also be the cause. Clinically, there is atrophy of the hypothenar and interossei muscles, causing the typical "claw hand" as well as a loss of sensation to touch and pain in the volar aspect of the little finger and medial half of the ring finger. The diagnosis is established by nerve conduction velocity studies. Treatment by translocation of the ulnar nerve at the elbow or surgical decompression in the cubital tunnel is usually successful. The ulnar nerve also may be entrapped at Guyon's canal in the wrist; in this case, surgical decompression is helpful.

Peroneal neuropathy: Peroneal neuropathy results from trauma or pressure around the knee (particularly from crossing the legs for a long period of time). Clinically, there is a foot drop, steppage gait of the involved leg, and loss of sensation to touch and pain in the dorsum of the foot and lower anterior aspect of the leg. Achilles reflexes are preserved. The straight leg–raising test is negative, and usually there is no history of low back pain. Nerve conduction velocity studies will confirm the diagnosis. Treatment is supportive, as spontaneous recovery is the rule rather than the exception.

Lateral femoral cutaneous neuropathy (meralgia paresthetica): The lateral femoral cutaneous nerve may be compressed as it passes beneath the inguinal ligament, especially in obese women who are pregnant and in lumbar lordosis. As a result, there is pain, paresthesia, and loss of sensation in the lateral thigh. Diabetics are especially prone to this disorder. In the differential diagnosis, a herniated disc at L2-L3 or L3-L4 must be ruled out. Nerve conduction velocity studies and electromyogram are usually normal. Treatment is supportive, as recovery is usually spontaneous.

Tarsal tunnel syndrome: Tarsal tunnel syndrome is caused by entrapment of the posterior tibial nerve as it passes beneath the flexor retinaculum located below and behind the medial malleolus. Patients experience burning, numbness, and tingling of the feet, especially at night. There may be hypesthesia and hypalgesia in the distribution of the lateral or medial plantar nerves. There is sensitivity over the tarsal tunnel, and the application of pressure there duplicates the symptoms. Nerve conduction velocity studies show prolonged distal latencies in the medial or lateral plantar nerve. Treatment with injection of corticosteroids and lidocaine into the tunnel will usually be successful, but the patient should be fitted with orthotics to prevent recurrences. Surgery is necessary in intractable cases.

Reflex sympathetic dystrophy: Reflex sympathetic dystrophy usually results from trauma to the neck and shoulder but may be associated with stroke, myocardial infarction, cervical spondylosis, and a number of other conditions. Initially, there is diffuse, nondermatomal pain of the shoulder and upper extremity, followed by edema and dystrophic skin and nail changes months later. Eventually, there may be diffuse atrophy of the extremity. Diagnosis is established by ruling out other forms of neuropathy, finding the underlying cause, and blocking the stellate ganglion. Treatment initially is conservative, with physiotherapy and stellate ganglion block. If these therapies fail, surgery may be necessary. Fortunately, most patients recover.

Other focal neuropathies of the trunk and extremities: Radial neuropathy, obturator neuropathy, femoral neuropathy, sciatic neuritis, and other neuropathies are sufficiently rare that the reader is referred to standard textbooks of neurology for their diagnosis and management.

MUSCULAR DYSTROPHY (CASE 1)

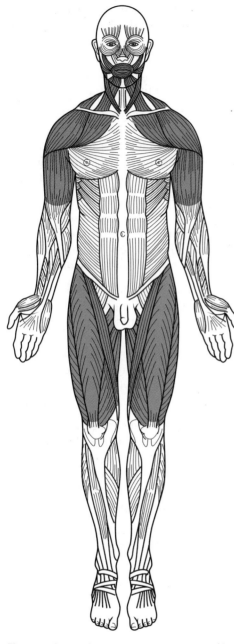

Figure 1. Spinal Cord: Muscular Dystrophy (Case 1)

A 14-year-old boy presented for examination because his friends teased him about the way his shoulders "stuck out in the back." Further questioning revealed that for the past year, he had noted weakness in his arms and legs, which worsened to the point that he was forced to drop out of the swim team. His uncle had died at an early age from a muscular disease.

Neurologic examination revealed tapir lips, pole neck, symmetric weakness, and atrophy of the muscles of the shoulder girdle, hips, and thighs. The patient had a waddling gait and a definite pelvic tilt. A muscle biopsy confirmed the diagnosis.

Treatable Diseases to Be Ruled Out
Peripheral neuropathy
Myasthenia gravis
Hypothyroid myopathy
Polymyositis

Comment: The anatomic profile demonstrates the involvement of the muscles, particularly the proximal muscles of the extremities.

Synopsis: Muscular dystrophy is an uncommon hereditary disorder of childhood and early adolescence. It presents in a variety of ways, most commonly as Duchenne's muscular dystrophy, myotonic dystrophy, or facioscapulohumeral dystrophy, as in the case presented here. The course usually is progressively downhill, with death due to respiratory failure in the second to fifth decade. Diagnostic workup should include routine complete blood count, urinalysis, and chemistry panel; a thyroid profile to exclude hypothyroidism; electromyography; and muscle biopsy. The electromyogram shows spontaneous fibrillations, positive sharp waves, and polyphasic action potentials. The muscle biopsy shows a variation in size of muscle bundles, necrosis, an increased number of central nuclei, and dystrophin-deficient tissue. Serum creatine kinase is elevated in most cases. There is no known cure for muscular dystrophy, but prednisone (0.15 to 0.75 mg/kg/day) improves muscle strength in Duchenne's muscular dystrophy.

MUSCULAR DYSTROPHY (CASE 2)

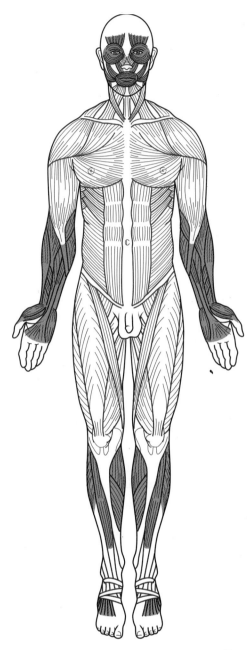

A 40-year-old white man presented with distal weakness of all four extremities, facial weakness, and dysarthria of several months' duration.

Neurologic examination revealed bilateral ptosis; a "hatchet face," depicting the facial weakness; weakness on flexion and extension of the hands, fingers, feet, and toes; distal atrophy of the muscles of the extremities; slow relaxation of the hand grip; and myotonia of the thenar eminence and tongue. In addition, the patient demonstrated premature baldness, cataracts, and testicular atrophy. The diagnosis was confirmed by electromyography and muscle biopsy.

Treatable Diseases to Be Ruled Out

Peripheral neuropathy
Myasthenia gravis
Hypothyroid myopathy
Polymyositis

Comment: The illustration shows the muscles involved in the disease. This is a typical case of myotonic dystrophy, as evidenced by the myotonia, premature baldness, cataracts, and testicular atrophy.

Synopsis: See page 100.

Figure 2. Spinal Cord: Muscular Dystrophy (Case 2)

MULTIPLE SCLEROSIS (CASE 1)

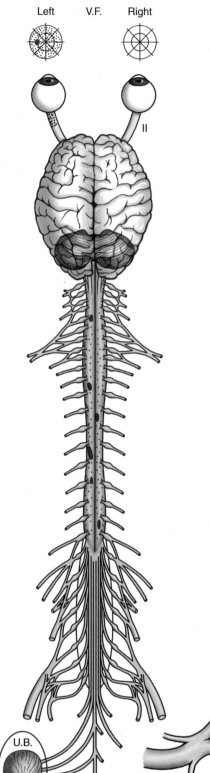

A 32-year-old white woman complained of intermittent weakness in her left arm and leg of 1 year's duration. This symptom cleared up almost completely 2 months prior to presentation, only to be followed by weakness in her left leg. For 3 months prior to presentation, she experienced incontinence of urine. At age 18, she had an episode of diplopia that cleared up spontaneously.

Neurologic examination revealed temporal pallor of the left optic disc, weakness of the left hand grip, and hyperactive reflexes in the left extremities. There was loss of superficial abdominal reflexes and a left Babinski sign. Her gait was hemiplegic. An MRI helped confirm the diagnosis.

Treatable Diseases to Be Ruled Out
Pernicious anemia
Spinal cord tumor
Neurosyphilis
Cervical spondylosis
Tuberculosis of the spine
Nutritional neuropathy

Comment: The illustration shows the involvement of the pyramidal tracts in an asymmetric fashion causing the left-sided weakness, hyperactive reflexes, and Babinski signs. Also illustrated is the optic nerve involvement and neurogenic bladder.

Synopsis: Multiple sclerosis is a demyelination disorder of the nervous system that in the majority of cases is characterized by exacerbation and remission over a long period of time. The etiology is unknown but is thought to be autoimmune in nature. The autoimmune reaction is directed against myelin antigen-specific T cells, but no specific antigen has been identified. Some cases of multiple sclerosis present with an acute transverse myelitis and optic neuritis (Devic disease, case 2), whereas others present as a slowly progressive downhill course of spastic paraplegia, mimicking a degenerative disease of the nervous system, such as primary lateral sclerosis. Multiple sclerosis may affect any area of the nervous system and may present in a variety of ways. Diagnosis is still clinical but can be confirmed by MRI findings of multiple demyelination plaques in various parts of the nervous system, especially when these findings correlate with the clinical picture. The findings of myelin basic protein and IgG oligoclonal bands in the spinal fluid are also helpful. Finally, visual, auditory, and somatosensory evoked potentials are positive in 60% to 80% of multiple sclerosis patients. Treatment includes high-dose intravenous corticosteroids for acute exacerbations and oral corticosteroids, immunosuppressant therapy, and interferon-β to prevent exacerbations (see Appendix C). Muscle spasticity may be treated with ba-

Figure 3. Spinal Cord: Multiple Sclerosis (Case 1)

clofen (up to 120 mg daily); dantrolene sodium, clonazepam, and tizanidine have also been effective. Supportive measures include physiotherapy, antidepressants, antiepileptic drugs for pain control, cholinergic and anticholinergic drugs for bladder dysfunction, and sildenafil citrate for sexual dysfunction.

MULTIPLE SCLEROSIS (CASE 2)

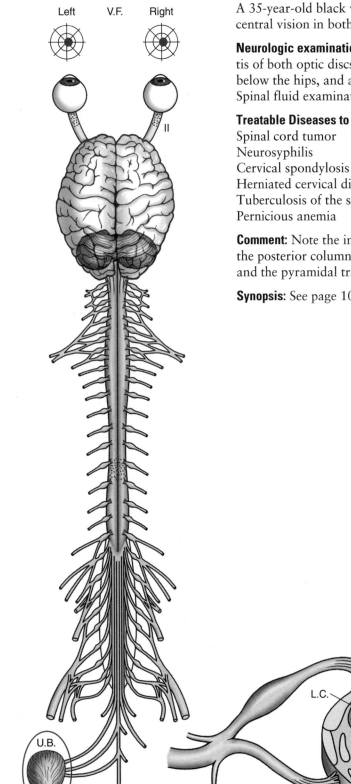

A 35-year-old black woman experienced sudden onset of staggering gait and loss of central vision in both eyes.

Neurologic examination 2 days later disclosed large bilateral central scotomata, papillitis of both optic discs, bilateral Babinski signs, loss of vibratory and position senses below the hips, and an ataxic gait. The bladder was percussed above the umbilicus. Spinal fluid examination revealed an elevated myelin basic protein.

Treatable Diseases to Be Ruled Out
Spinal cord tumor
Neurosyphilis
Cervical spondylosis
Herniated cervical disc
Tuberculosis of the spine
Pernicious anemia

Comment: Note the involvement of the optic nerves, producing the central scotomata; the posterior column, producing the loss of vibratory and position senses and ataxia; and the pyramidal tracts, causing Babinski signs and neurogenic bladder.

Synopsis: See page 102.

Figure 4. Spinal Cord: Multiple Sclerosis (Case 2)

MULTIPLE SCLEROSIS (CASE 3)

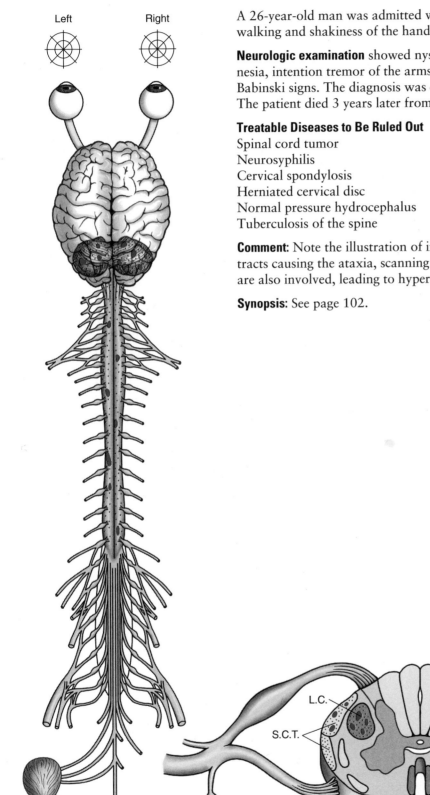

A 26-year-old man was admitted with a 3-year history of intermittent difficulty in walking and shakiness of the hands.

Neurologic examination showed nystagmus, scanning speech, bilateral dysdiadochokinesia, intention tremor of the arms and legs, ataxia, hyperactive reflexes, and bilateral Babinski signs. The diagnosis was confirmed by an MRI of the brain and spinal cord. The patient died 3 years later from a renal infection.

Treatable Diseases to Be Ruled Out
Spinal cord tumor
Neurosyphilis
Cervical spondylosis
Herniated cervical disc
Normal pressure hydrocephalus
Tuberculosis of the spine

Comment: Note the illustration of involvement of the cerebellum and spinocerebellar tracts causing the ataxia, scanning speech, and intention tremor. The lateral columns are also involved, leading to hyperactive reflexes and Babinski signs.

Synopsis: See page 102.

Figure 5. Spinal Cord: Multiple Sclerosis (Case 3)

NUTRITIONAL NEUROPATHY

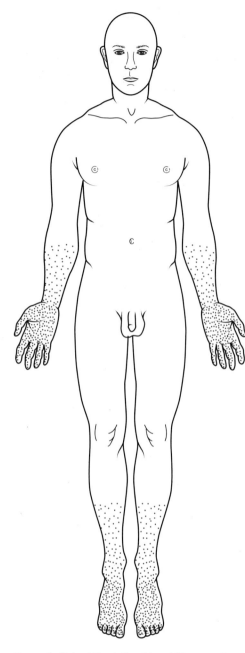

A 54-year-old white man underwent a subtotal gastrectomy for a peptic ulcer. His postoperative course was stormy, and oral intake was poor for the first month. Approximately 5 weeks after surgery, he suddenly developed weakness in all four extremities and loss of feeling in both hands.

Neurologic examination revealed marked weakness, atrophy, and diminished deep tendon reflexes in all four extremities; glove and stocking hypesthesia and hypalgesia; almost total loss of vibratory sense below the knees; and a high-stepping gait. After a week of thiamine and multivitamin supplements, the patient's symptoms and signs improved remarkably.

Treatable Diseases to Be Ruled Out
Infectious polyneuritis
Lead neuropathy
Pernicious anemia
Polymyositis

Comment: The illustration demonstrates the glove and stocking hypesthesia and hypalgesia.

Synopsis: This case illustrates the typical presentation of nutritional neuropathy. The disorder is often associated with alcoholism, poor diet, malabsorption syndrome, anorexia nervosa, and bulimia. Diagnosis is usually made from the clinical picture and response to therapy. However, the red blood cell transketolase activity is often decreased whereas serum pyruvate and lactate are increased, providing confirmation of the clinical impression. Unfortunately, these tests often are not available. Nerve conduction velocity is routinely decreased. Treatment is with large doses of B vitamin and multivitamin supplements, as outlined in Appendix C. Prognosis is good if treatment is instituted early.

Figure 1. Spinal Cord: Nutritional Neuropathy

PERONEAL MUSCULAR ATROPHY

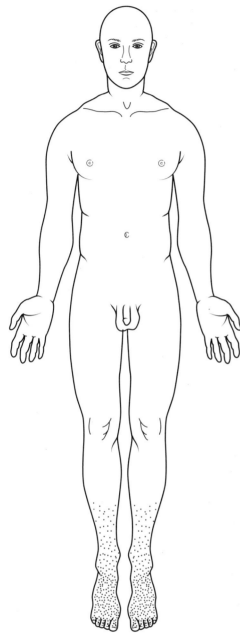

A 16-year-old white boy complained of dragging his feet and "skinny legs" for the past 8 months. His father died in his 30s of a similar condition.

Neurologic examination revealed weakness and atrophy of the lower legs, with bilateral footdrop; stocking hypalgesia and hypesthesia; absence of Achilles reflexes; and a steppage gait. Orthopedic evaluation revealed pes cavus and hammer toes bilaterally. Nerve conduction velocities were uniformly decreased in the lower extremities.

Treatable Diseases to Be Ruled Out
Nutritional neuropathy
Cauda equina tumor
Lead neuropathy
Herniated disc

Comment: The illustration shows the stocking hypesthesia and hypalgesia.

Synopsis: Peroneal muscular atrophy is an inherited disorder and an autosomal dominant trait in most cases. At least three specific gene abnormalities have been identified. Most cases begin between the second and fourth decades. The most useful diagnostic test is the finding of identical features in family members. Nerve conduction velocity studies and sural nerve biopsy can confirm the diagnosis. There is no specific treatment. An orthopedic consultation is helpful for supportive care of the feet.

Figure 1. Spinal Cord: Peroneal Muscular Atrophy

POLIOMYELITIS

Left   Right

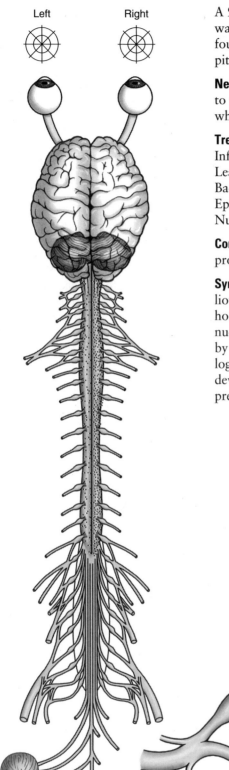

A 9-year-old white girl had a sudden onset of diarrhea, vomiting, and fever, which was diagnosed as viral gastroenteritis. Four days later, she became drowsy and was found to have flaccid paralysis in her right arm and leg. She was admitted to the hospital with a diagnosis of cerebrovascular accident.

Neurologic examination revealed hypoactive reflexes in all four extremities in addition to profound weakness of the right extremities. Spinal fluid examination revealed 310 white cells/mm^3 and an opening pressure of 280 mm H_2O.

Treatable Diseases to Be Ruled Out
Infectious polyneuritis
Lead neuropathy
Bacterial meningitis
Epidural abscess
Nutritional neuropathy

Comment: Note the involvement of the anterior horn cells in an asymmetric fashion, producing the right-sided weakness and diffuse hypoactive reflexes.

Synopsis: Poliomyelitis is an infectious disease produced by three types of polioviruses. Because of excellent vaccines, the disease is rarely seen today. The anterior horn cells are involved in the spinal cord and brainstem, but the extraocular muscle nuclei are spared. Only 10% of cases are associated with paralysis. Diagnosis is made by the spinal fluid leukocytosis and clinical picture, although viral isolation and serologic tests may be done. Treatment is supportive, as there is no cure. A few patients develop a postpolio syndrome 20 to 30 years later, with progressive weakness of the previously involved muscle; there is no specific treatment for this complication.

V.H.

Figure 2. Spinal Cord: Poliomyelitis

PORPHYRIA

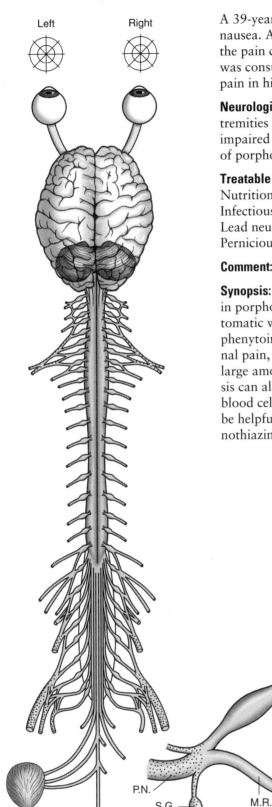

Left   Right

A 39-year-old white man had an episode of colicky right lower quadrant pain and nausea. An appendectomy was performed. The appendix was reported normal, and the pain continued postoperatively. Two weeks after hospitalization, a neurologist was consulted because the patient had become delirious and complained of severe pain in his arms and legs.

Neurologic examination revealed weakness and atrophy of the muscles in all four extremities and mild tenderness of the peripheral nerve trunks. Mental status showed impaired judgment and lack of emotional control. Urinalysis revealed large amounts of porphobilinogen.

Treatable Diseases to Be Ruled Out
Nutritional neuropathy
Infectious polyneuritis
Lead neuropathy and encephalopathy
Pernicious anemia

Comment: The illustration shows the symmetric involvement of the peripheral nerves.

Synopsis: Porphyria is a hereditary disorder that usually results from a 50% deficiency in porphobilinogen deaminase. Patients are usually asymptomatic but become symptomatic when treated with drugs such as barbiturates, sulfonamide, estrogen, and phenytoin. The clinical picture presented here is typical and includes colicky abdominal pain, motor neuropathy, and encephalopathy. Diagnosis is established by finding large amounts of porphobilinogen or γ-aminolevulinic acid in the urine. The diagnosis can also be made by finding a deficiency of uroporphyrinogen I synthetase in red blood cells. Treatment with intravenous dextrose or hematin (see Appendix C) may be helpful. Propranolol is useful to treat the tachycardia and hypertension. The phenothiazines may control the mental symptoms. Prognosis is good for recovery.

S.R.

P.N.

S.G.

M.R.

Figure 3. Spinal Cord: Porphyria

PERIARTERITIS NODOSA

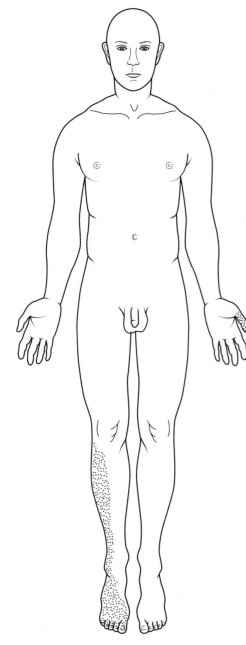

A 37-year-old white man had a sudden attack of abdominal pain and distention. Exploratory laparotomy revealed a mesenteric artery thrombosis. Four days after surgery, he developed a wristdrop and right footdrop.

Neurologic examination revealed hypesthesia and hypalgesia in the distribution of the left radial and right common peroneal nerves. A muscle biopsy confirmed the diagnosis.

Treatable Diseases to Be Ruled Out
Nutritional neuropathy
Lead neuropathy
Other collagen diseases

Comment: The illustration shows the sensory loss in the left radial and right peroneal nerve contribution.

Synopsis: This is a case of mononeuritis multiplex, which is typically associated with collagen diseases such as periarteritis nodosa, lupus erythematosus (SLE), rheumatoid arthritis, and giant cell arteritis. Diagnosis is usually confirmed by a positive antinuclear antibody titer, positive double-strand DNA, or muscle biopsy. If doubt still exists after these studies, sural nerve biopsy may be required. Treatment with corticosteroids (see Appendix C for dosages and schedules) is usually effective for most collagen diseases, but intravenous cyclophosphamide has been effective in SLE.

Figure 4. Spinal Cord: Periarteritis Nodosa

PERNICIOUS ANEMIA

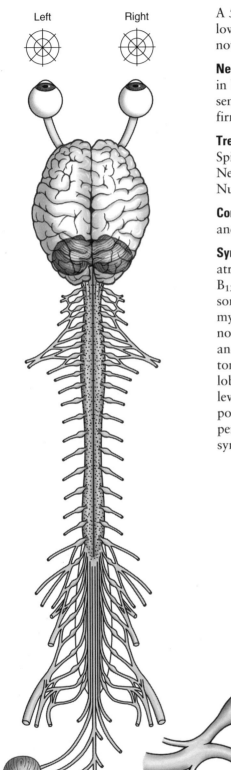

A 53-year-old white man had increasing weakness, numbness, and tingling in his lower extremities associated with difficulty walking for the past 6 months. He also noted difficulty remembering names, numbers, and faces for several months.

Neurologic examination revealed pallor of the nails and mucous membranes, weakness in both lower extremities, bilateral Babinski signs, and loss of vibratory and position senses below the waist. Serum vitamin B_{12} level was decreased. The Schilling test confirmed the diagnosis.

Treatable Diseases to Be Ruled Out
Spinal cord tumor
Neurosyphilis
Nutritional neuropathy

Comment: Note the involvement of the posterior columns, causing the loss of vibratory and position senses, and the lateral columns, causing the Babinski signs and weakness.

Synopsis: Pernicious anemia is usually the result of vitamin B_{12} deficiency caused by atrophy of the gastric mucosa and depletion of intrinsic factor, which is important for B_{12} absorption. However, B_{12} deficiency may result from dietary deficiency, malabsorption syndrome, drugs, and a variety of other causes. Without vitamin B_{12}, the myelin in the brain and spinal cord deteriorate, leading to the symptoms and signs noted above. It is not usually appreciated that these patients may have memory loss and other neuropsychiatric symptoms; indeed, these may be the only presenting symptoms in many cases. The diagnosis is established by a hemogram that shows megaloblastic anemia and a low serum vitamin B_{12} level with a normal serum folic acid level. The Schilling test will confirm that the lack of intrinsic factor is the cause of poor B_{12} absorption. Treatment with vitamin B_{12} intramuscularly, as outlined in Appendix C, will bring complete resolution in most cases, although the neuropsychiatric symptoms may take months to resolve.

P.C.

L.C.

Figure 5. Spinal Cord: Pernicious Anemia

SPINAL CORD TUMOR (CASE 1)
(Brown–Séquard Syndrome)

Left   Right

A 35-year-old black woman who was admitted to the hospital had complained of pain in her left breast and weakness in her left leg for the past year. Six months before admission, she was told at another clinic that she had multiple sclerosis. One month before admission, she experienced incontinence of urine.

Neurologic examination revealed weakness, spasticity, increased reflexes, and ankle clonus in the left leg. Vibratory and position senses were lost below the hip on the left side, and pain and temperature were lost below T6 on the right. Spinal fluid examination revealed a total protein of 220 mg/dL. An MRI of the thoracic spine established the diagnosis.

Treatable Diseases to Be Ruled Out
Epidural abscess
Epidural hematoma
Herniated disc

Comment: The illustration shows the tumor compressing the dorsal root and left half of the spinal cord, causing loss of vibratory and position senses on the homolateral side of the lesion and loss of pain and temperature senses on the contralateral side of the lesion.

Synopsis: The most common benign tumors of the spinal cord are meningiomas and neurofibromas. These tumors usually present as an extramedullary mass (cases 1 and 2), whereas ependymomas and gliomas present as an intramedullary lesion (case 3). Metastatic tumors from the prostate (case 4), breast, and lung also may present as an extramedullary lesion. One should also look for lymphoma or multiple myeloma when a patient presents with signs of root and cord compression. MRI is the diagnostic procedure of choice, and combined CT and myelography may help with localization. Spinal fluid examination is rarely necessary to pin down the diagnosis. Surgical treatment is often successful for cord decompression. The prognosis for benign tumors is good.

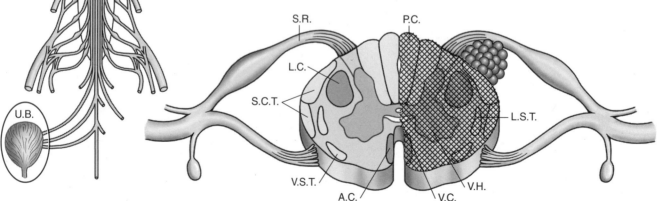

Figure 1. Spinal Cord: Spinal Cord Tumor (Case 1, Brown-Séquard Syndrome)

SPINAL CORD TUMOR (CASE 2)
(Cauda Equina Tumor)

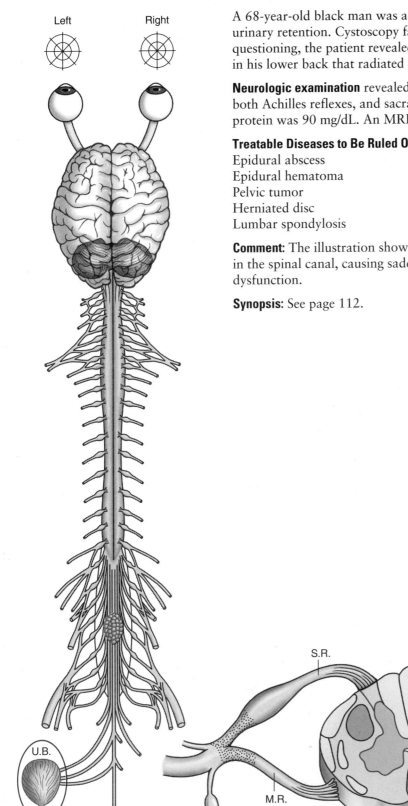

A 68-year-old black man was admitted to the urology service because of chronic urinary retention. Cystoscopy failed to disclose bladder neck obstruction. On careful questioning, the patient revealed that in the past year, he had experienced severe pain in his lower back that radiated down his left leg.

Neurologic examination revealed a positive straight leg–raising test bilaterally, loss of both Achilles reflexes, and sacral anesthesia and analgesia. The spinal fluid total protein was 90 mg/dL. An MRI of the lumbosacral spine confirmed the diagnosis.

Treatable Diseases to Be Ruled Out
Epidural abscess
Epidural hematoma
Pelvic tumor
Herniated disc
Lumbar spondylosis

Comment: The illustration shows the tumor compressing the lumbosacral nerve roots in the spinal canal, causing saddle anesthesia and analgesia along with bladder dysfunction.

Synopsis: See page 112.

Figure 2. Spinal Cord: Spinal Cord Tumor (Case 2, Cauda Equina Tumor)

SPINAL CORD TUMOR (CASE 3)
(Intramedullary Tumor)

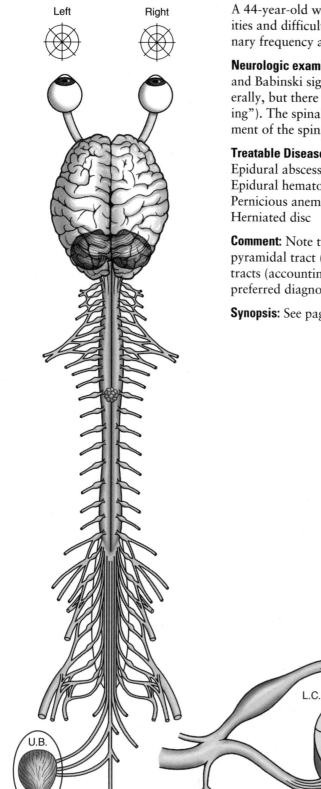

Left   Right

A 44-year-old white woman complained of progressive weakness in her lower extremities and difficulty walking for the past 8 months. For the past 3 months, she had urinary frequency and urgency.

Neurologic examination disclosed weakness, spasticity, increased deep tendon reflexes, and Babinski signs in both lower extremities. A sensory level was located at T4 bilaterally, but there was no loss of pain or temperature sense below L5 ("sacral sparing"). The spinal fluid total protein was 140 mg/dL. A myelogram revealed enlargement of the spinal cord at T3 and T4, but there was no block.

Treatable Diseases to Be Ruled Out
Epidural abscess
Epidural hematoma
Pernicious anemia
Herniated disc

Comment: Note the central location of the tumor, with outward compression of the pyramidal tract (explaining the weakness and spasticity) and lateral spinothalamic tracts (accounting for the bilateral loss of pain and temperature senses). MRI is the preferred diagnostic study.

Synopsis: See page 112.

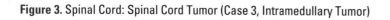

Figure 3. Spinal Cord: Spinal Cord Tumor (Case 3, Intramedullary Tumor)

SPINAL CORD TUMOR (CASE 4)
(Metastatic Carcinoma)

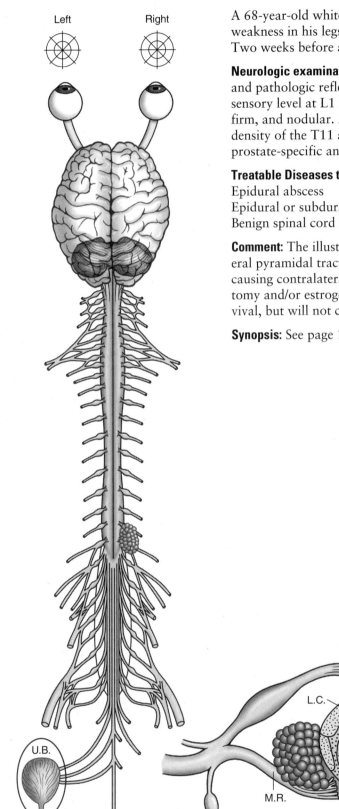

Left   Right

A 68-year-old white man with a 1-year history of back pain developed progressive weakness in his legs and difficulty walking 3 months before admission to the hospital. Two weeks before admission, he became incontinent of urine and feces.

Neurologic examination revealed weakness, spasticity, increased deep tendon reflexes, and pathologic reflexes in both lower extremities; a short-stepped, spastic gait; and a sensory level at L1 on the left side. On rectal examination, the prostate was large, firm, and nodular. A roentgenogram of the lower thoracic spine revealed increased density of the T11 and T12 vertebrae. Laboratory examination revealed elevated prostate-specific antigen and both acid and alkaline phosphatase.

Treatable Diseases to Be Ruled Out
Epidural abscess
Epidural or subdural hematoma
Benign spinal cord tumor

Comment: The illustration shows the tumor compressing the spinal cord, causing bilateral pyramidal tract signs, and involvement of the right lateral spinothalamic tract, causing contralateral loss of pain and temperature senses. Treatment with orchiectomy and/or estrogen and luteinizing hormone-releasing hormone may prolong survival, but will not cure the disease. The same holds true for radiation.

Synopsis: See page 112.

U.B.

L.C.

S.C.T.

L.S.T.

M.R.

Figure 4. Spinal Cord: Spinal Cord Tumor (Case 4, Metastatic Carcinoma)

SYPHILITIC MENINGOMYELITIS

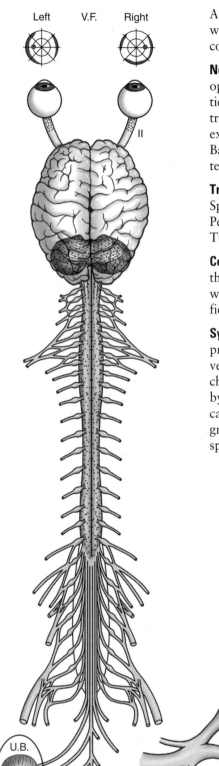

Left V.F. Right

II

U.B.

A 51-year-old horse trainer experienced increasing weakness in his legs and difficulty walking for the past 6 months. His sight had been failing for the past year, and he complained of the inability to "hold his water." He denied a history of lues.

Neurologic examination revealed pallor and an increase of cribriform markings in both optic discs, concentric narrowing of the visual fields, and loss of visual acuity. The patient's speech was slow and dysarthric. In the extremities, he exhibited an intention tremor on finger-to-nose and heel-to-knee tests bilaterally, weakness of flexion and extension of the toes and feet, hyperactive patellar and Achilles reflexes, and bilateral Babinski signs. Results of fluorescent treponemal antibody absorption (FTA-ABS) testing of the spinal fluid were positive.

Treatable Diseases to Be Ruled Out
Spinal cord tumor
Pernicious anemia
Tuberculosis of the spinal column

Comment: Note the involvement of the spinocerebellar tracts and cerebellum, causing the intention tremor and dysarthria; the pyramidal tracts, causing the spasticity and weakness of the lower extremities and Babinski signs; and the optic nerve, causing the field defects.

Synopsis: Syphilitic meningomyelitis, a form of neurosyphilis rarely seen today, may produce a progressive paraplegia. Syphilis may also cause tabes dorsalis, acute transverse myelitis, meningitis, and amyotrophic lateral sclerosis syndrome, as well as chronic pachymeningitis, particularly in the cervical region. Diagnosis is established by serologic tests of the blood and spinal fluid, especially the FTA-ABS test, as in this case. Treatment with penicillin, as outlined in Appendix C, will usually halt the progression of this disease, and may cure it. Surgery may be necessary to decompress the spinal cord.

L.C.

S.C.T.

Figure 5. Syphilitic Meningomyelitis

SYRINGOMYELIA

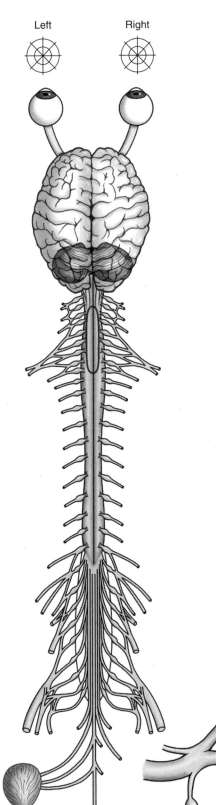

Left   Right

A 54-year-old bookkeeper with a long-standing history of syringomyelia complained of progressive weakness in his right hand. He returned for examination because he feared losing his job.

Neurologic examination revealed weakness, atrophy, and fasciculations of the interossei, thenar, and hypothenar muscles of both hands; atrophy of both shoulder girdles; and loss of pain and temperature senses between the C2 and T6 dermatomes bilaterally. Deep tendon reflexes were increased in the lower extremities, and there was impairment of vibratory and position senses below the knees. An MRI confirmed the diagnosis.

Treatable Diseases to Be Ruled Out
Spinal cord tumor
Cervical spondylosis
Herniated disc
Bilateral cervical ribs
Nutritional neuropathy
Ulnar entrapment syndrome

Comment: The cavity creates pressure on the ventral commissure and lateral spinothalamic tracts, causing loss of pain and temperature senses; on the anterior horn cells, causing atrophy and fasciculations; on the pyramidal tracts, causing hyperactive reflexes and weakness in the lower extremities; and on the posterior columns, causing loss of vibratory and position senses.

Synopsis: Syringomyelia is a rare, slowly progressive neurologic disease that may present as a lobular dilatation of the central canal or a cavity that has no connection with the central canal. The latter type is usually post-traumatic or related to hemorrhage, ischemia, or radiation necrosis of the spinal cord. The diagnosis is made by MRI or single-photon emission tomography. A small syrinx may be left untreated, but if symptoms and signs progress, a neurosurgeon should be consulted for decompression or a shunting procedure, which may occasionally retard the progression.

P.C.

L.C.

L.S.T.

V.H.

V.C.

Figure 6. Syringomyelia

TABES DORSALIS

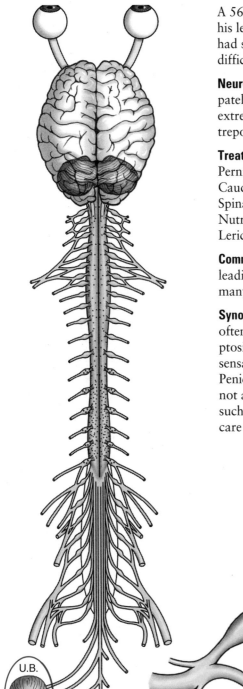

A 56-year-old black man was treated by his primary physician for shooting pain in his legs and enlargement of his knee joints for the past 2 years. He was told that he had severe arthritis. Two months before admission to the hospital, he developed difficulty walking in the dark.

Neurologic examination disclosed Argyll Robertson pupils, Charcot joints, absent patellar and Achilles reflexes, loss of position and vibratory senses in the lower extremities, and a wide-based ataxic gait. Blood and spinal fluid fluorescent treponemal antibody absorption tests were positive.

Treatable Diseases to Be Ruled Out
Pernicious anemia
Cauda equina tumor
Spinal stenosis
Nutritional neuropathy
Leriche syndrome

Comment: Note the involvement of the dorsal columns and sensory nerve roots, leading to the shooting pains, loss of vibratory and position senses, and ataxic gait. In many cases, bladder retention is also present.

Synopsis: Tabes dorsalis is a rare form of tertiary syphilis, but it may be seen more often in undeveloped countries. Frequently, associated optic atrophy and bilateral ptosis are present. Trophic ulcers may occur in the feet as a result of the loss of sensation. Diagnosis is best made by serologic tests of the blood and spinal fluid. Penicillin therapy, as outlined in Appendix C, will wipe out the spirochetes but may not afford much of a cure. The lightning pains may be helped by antiepileptic drugs such as phenytoin or carbamazepine. An orthopedic surgeon should be consulted for care of the Charcot joints. Test for HIV in all cases.

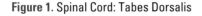

Figure 1. Spinal Cord: Tabes Dorsalis

THORACIC OUTLET SYNDROME

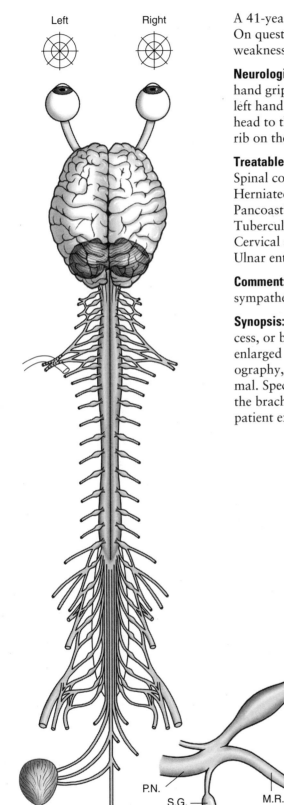

Left   Right

A 41-year-old white man complained of a drooping left eyelid of 2 weeks' duration. On questioning, it was discovered that he had intermittent pain, numbness, and weakness in his left arm for the past 10 years.

Neurologic examination revealed a left-sided Horner syndrome, weakness of the left hand grip, diminished left triceps reflex, and mild atrophy of the small muscles of the left hand. The left radial pulse was obliterated by hyperextension and rotation of the head to the left (Adson's test). A radiograph of the cervical spine revealed a cervical rib on the left side.

Treatable Diseases to Be Ruled Out
Spinal cord tumor
Herniated cervical disc
Pancoast's tumor
Tuberculosis of the spine
Cervical spondylosis
Ulnar entrapment syndrome

Comment: The illustration shows the cervical rib compressing the brachial plexus and sympathetic ganglia.

Synopsis: Thoracic outlet syndrome may be caused by a cervical rib, transverse process, or band arising from the seventh cervical vertebra. It may also be caused by an enlarged scalenus anticus muscle. Diagnosis can be confirmed by radiography, arteriography, and electromyography. Nerve conduction velocity studies are usually normal. Specific treatment is by surgical removal of the cervical rib or decompression of the brachial plexus. However, many cases can be treated conservatively by having the patient exercise the trapezius muscles (shoulder shrugs) or improve posture.

P.N.

S.G.

M.R.

Rib

Figure 2. Spinal Cord: Thoracic Outlet Syndrome

Key to Master Diagram of the Brain

I	Olfactory bulb
II	Optic nerve
III	Oculomotor nerve
IV	Trochlear nerve
V	Trigeminal nerve
V_1	Ophthalmic division of trigeminal nerve
V_2	Maxillary division of trigeminal nerve
VI	Abducens nerve
VII	Facial nerve
c. VIII	Cochlear nerve
v. VIII	Vestibular nerve
IX	Glossopharyngeal nerve
X	Vagus nerve
XI	Spinal accessory nerve
XII	Hypoglossus nerve

A.C.	Anterior communicating artery
A.C.A.	Anterior cerebral artery
A.N.	Ambiguus nucleus
A.S.	Aqueduct of Sylvius
A.S.A.	Anterior spinal artery
B.A.	Basilar artery
B.C.	Brachium conjunctivum
B.P.C.	Basis pedunculi cerebri
C.C.	Corpus callosum
C.C.A.	Common carotid artery
C.H.	Cerebellar hemisphere
C.N.	Caudate nucleus
D.	Dura
D.C.N.	Dorsal cochlear nucleus
E.C.A.	External carotid artery
E.R.	External rectus muscle
F.L.	Frontal lobe
F.M.	Muscles supplied by facial nerve
G.F.	Genu of the facial nerve
G.P.	Globus pallidus
I.C.	Internal capsule
I.C.A.	Internal carotid artery
I.O.	Inferior olive
I.R.	Inferior rectus muscle
M.B.	Mammillary bodies
M.C.A.	Middle cerebellar artery
M.L.	Medial lemniscus
M.L.F.	Medial longitudinal fasciculus
M.R.	Medial rectus muscle
O.C.	Optic chiasma
O.L.	Occipital lobe
O.T.	Optic tract
P.	Putamen
P.A.G.	Periaqueductal gray
P.C.	Posterior communicating artery
P.C.A.	Posterior cerebellar artery
P.G.	Pituitary gland
P.I.C.A.	Posterior inferior cerebellar artery
P.T.	Pyramidal tract
R.B.	Restiform body
R.N.	Red nucleus
S.A.	Subclavian artery
S.N.	Substantia nigra
S.S.S.	Superior sagittal sinus
S.T.	Spinothalamic tract
S.T.V.	Spinal tract of trigeminal nerve
T.	Tongue
T.L.	Temporal lobe
V.A.	Vertebral artery
V.C.	Vermis cerebelli
V.C.N.	Ventral cochlear nucleus
V.F.	Visual fields
V.N.	Vestibular nuclei

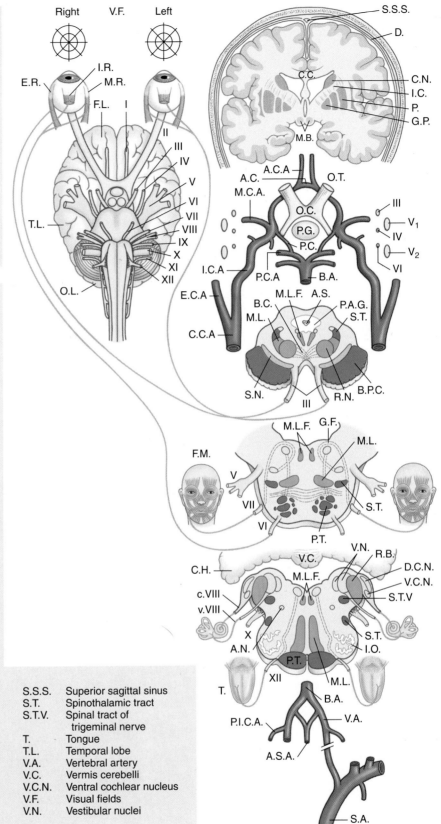

Diseases of the Brain and Brainstem

ACOUSTIC NEUROMA

A 58-year-old white woman has had a high-pitched ringing in her left ear for the past 5 years and a staggering gait for the past month.

Neurologic examination revealed nystagmus on the left lateral gaze, marked hearing loss in the left ear, and a wide-based ataxic gait. On Weber's test, sound lateralized to the right; Rinne test showed 2:1 air-to-bone conduction bilaterally. These findings indicated perceptive deafness on the left side. An MRI confirmed the diagnosis.

Treatable Diseases to Be Ruled Out
Neurosyphilis
Cholesteatoma
Foramen magnum tumor
Vertebral-basilar insufficiency
Petrositis
Cerebellar abscess
Tuberculous meningitis
Platybasia

Comment: The illustration shows the involvement of the cerebellum, causing the nystagmus and ataxia, and the acoustic nerve, causing the perceptive deafness.

Synopsis: Acoustic neuroma is a benign tumor arising from the Schwann cells of the vestibular nerve and constitutes 5% to 10% of all brain tumors. The tumor may extend to involve the fifth and seventh cranial nerves if it is not detected early. Diagnosis is best confirmed by gadolinium-enhanced MRI. Treatment is surgery. Prognosis is excellent if the tumor is detected early.

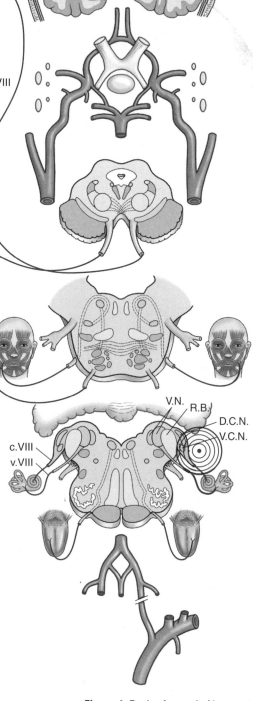

Figure 1. Brain: Acoustic Neuroma

ALZHEIMER'S DISEASE

A 65-year-old white woman was admitted to the hospital with a 3-year history of an insidious onset of forgetfulness and impaired judgment, with an occasional acute episode of disorientation. For 3 months before admission, she required assistance with activities of daily living and was incontinent of urine.

Neurologic examination revealed marked disorientation in time, place, and politics; mixed aphasia; apraxia; pathologic mouth opening reflexes; a grasp reflex on the right; and hyperactive reflexes of all extremities. An MRI showed diffuse dilation of the ventricles and enlargement of the sulci.

Treatable Diseases to Be Ruled Out
Space-occupying lesion
General paresis
Wernicke's encephalopathy
Toxic encephalopathy
Normal pressure hydrocephalus
Pernicious anemia

Comment: The illustration shows the diffusely enlarged ventricles and sulci and involvement throughout the cerebral cortex characteristic of Alzheimer's disease. This is in contrast to Pick's disease, which primarily affects the frontal and temporal lobes.

Synopsis: Alzheimer's disease is a diffuse, degenerative disorder of the cerebral cortex. The etiology is unknown, although a relationship to apolipoprotein E (Apo E) is being intensely investigated. The disease usually begins after 70 years of age, but 1% of patients develop the disorder between the ages of 50 and 70. Diagnosis is established by psychometric testing, MRI, or single-photon emission computed tomography, and other disorders are excluded by laboratory and special diagnostic tests. Treatment is symptomatic and supportive, although donepezil (Aricept; Pfizer, New York, NY) may improve cognition for a short period during the course of the disease. Prognosis is not good, and most patients die of infectious disease within 5 to 15 years after onset.

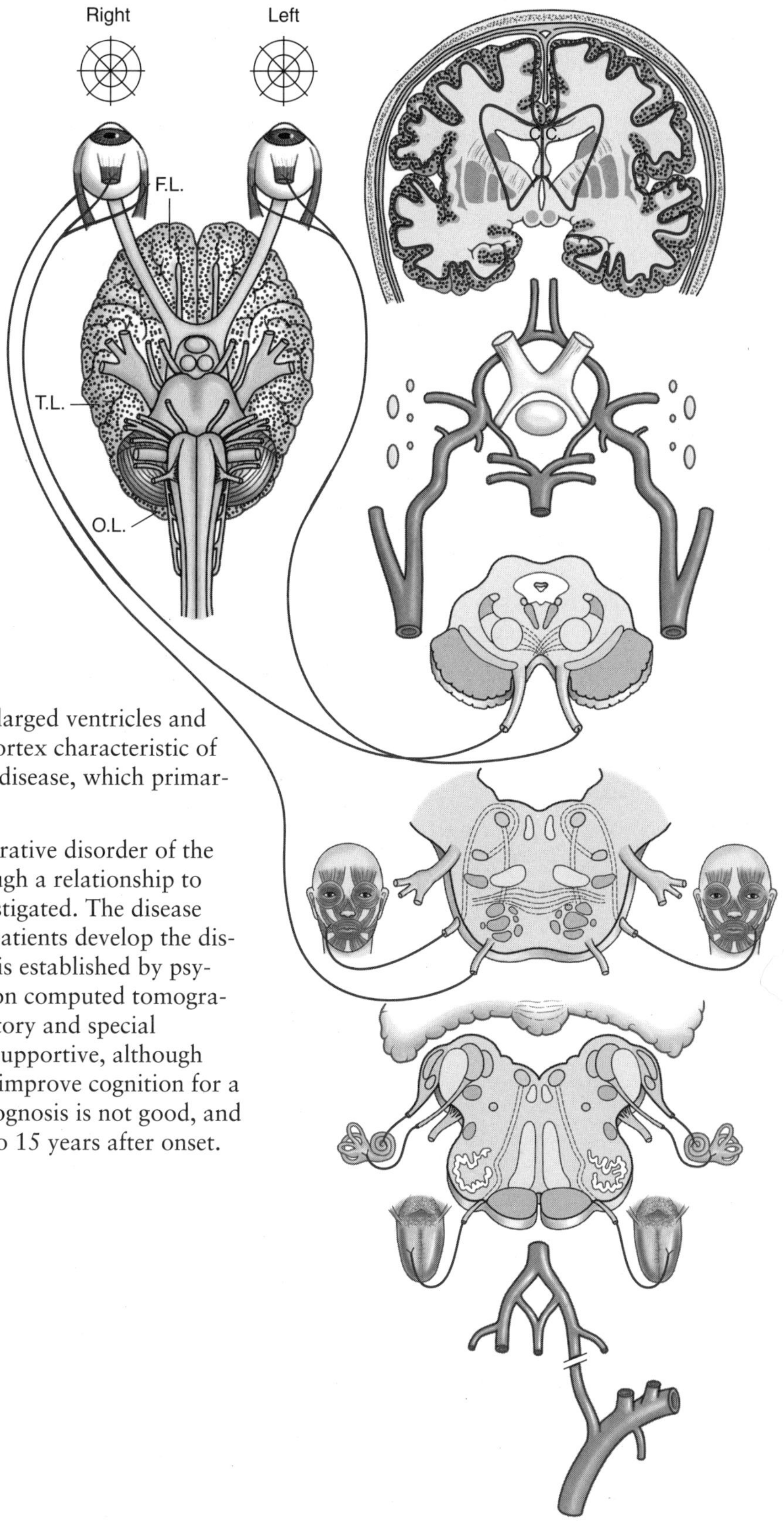

Figure 2. Brain: Alzheimer's Disease

AMYOTROPHIC LATERAL SCLEROSIS (BULBAR)

A 38-year-old trumpet player had difficulty positioning his lips to play for the past 2 months. He also had difficulty swallowing.

Neurologic examination revealed weakness, atrophy, and fasciculations bilaterally in the face, tongue, and sternocleidomastoid and trapezius muscles; bulbar speech; and hyperactive reflexes of all four extremities. Electromyography assisted in confirming the diagnosis. Other laboratory studies and radiographs were normal.

Treatable Diseases to Be Ruled Out

Brainstem neoplasm
Myasthenia gravis
Vertebral-basilar artery insufficiency
Neurosyphilis
Platybasia

Comment: The illustration shows the involvement of the corticospinal tracts, causing the hyperactive reflexes in the extremities, the facial nuclei causing weakness, atrophy and fasciculations of the facial muscles, and the hypoglossal nuclei, causing the atrophy and fasciculations of the tongue.

Synopsis: See page 85.

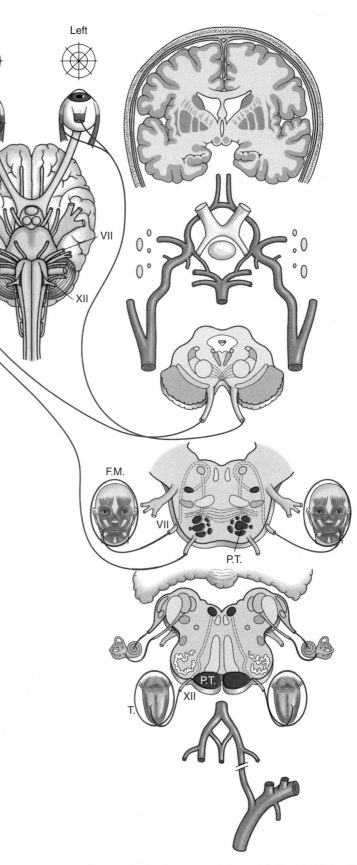

Figure 3. Brain: Amyotrophic Lateral Sclerosis (Bulbar)

ANTERIOR CEREBRAL ARTERY THROMBOSIS

A 59-year-old left-handed black woman gradually became unable to support her weight on her left leg, and she stumbled and fell.

Neurologic examination revealed a confused and disoriented patient with expressive aphasia; flaccid paralysis and diminished sensation to touch and vibration in the left leg; minimal weakness of the left hand and fingers; and a left-sided Babinski sign. A CT scan with enhancement revealed an ischemic infarct in the right frontal lobe. Angiography showed an occlusion of the right anterior cerebral artery but no large-vessel disease.

Treatable Diseases to Be Ruled Out
Cerebral embolism
Subdural hematoma
Carotid artery stenosis
Collagen disease
Blood dyscrasia

Comment: The illustration shows the infarction of the right parasagittal area, causing weakness and loss of sensation in the left lower extremity, and the occlusion of the anterior cerebral artery (*arrow*).

Synopsis: A thrombosis of the large cerebral arteries is usually associated with atherosclerosis; however, several factors predispose to thrombosis, including diabetes mellitus, hypertension, smoking, collagen disease, and blood dyscrasia. In contrast to cerebral embolism and hemorrhage, a cerebral thrombosis is more gradual in onset, as exemplified by this case, and headache and systemic symptoms are rarely present. Diagnosis is established by CT scan or MRI, but CT is better for excluding hemorrhage, especially if thrombolysis therapy is contemplated. If a cerebral embolism is suspected, the patient should be thoroughly investigated for myocardial infarction, subacute bacterial endocarditis, cardiac arrhythmia, and other cardiac causes of embolism. A carotid duplex scan should also be done. Treatment is usually supportive, but if the stroke is less than 3 hours old, thrombolysis therapy should be considered in consultation with a neurologist (see Appendix C). Stroke rehabilitation should begin immediately.

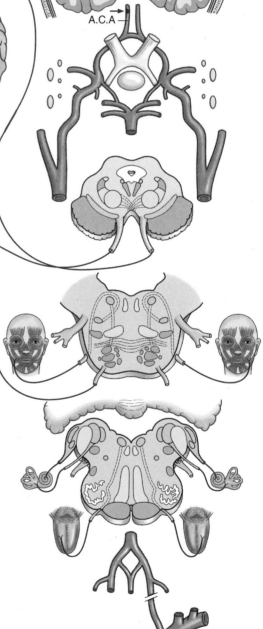

Figure 4. Brain: Anterior Cerebral Artery Thrombosis

BACTERIAL MENINIGITIS

A 9-year-old white boy developed a cough and sore throat 2 days before admission to the hospital. On the day of admission, he awoke with a severe headache, confusion, nausea, and vomiting.

Neurologic examination revealed a petechial rash of the extremities, nuchal rigidity, and Kernig's sign (resistance to extension of the legs at the knee) but no focal neurologic signs. Spinal fluid examination revealed an opening pressure of 260 mm H_2O; 1240 white blood cells/mL, mostly neutrophils; and decreased glucose and chloride. A culture was positive for *Neisseria meningitidis*.

Treatable Diseases to Be Ruled Out
Subarachnoid hemorrhage
Cavernous abscess
Retropharyngeal abscess

Comment: The illustration shows the diffuse involvement of the meninges causing the nuchal rigidity and Kernig's sign.

Synopsis: Meningococcal meningitis typically begins with invasion of the nasopharynx and subsequent hematogenous spread to the skin and meninges. The spread is rapid, as in this case. Other frequent causes of bacterial meningitis include *Streptococcus pneumoniae* and *Haemophilus influenzae*. The diagnosis is established by spinal tap. If there are possible focal neurologic findings or papilledema, a CT scan should be done before the spinal tap. Treatment is with antibiotics, particularly intravenous penicillin G, as outlined in Appendix C. The prognosis is good if treatment is begun early.

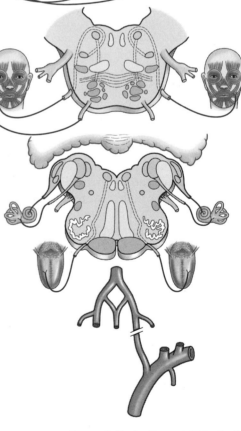

Figure 1. Brain: Bacterial Meningitis

BASILAR ARTERY THROMBOSIS

A 62-year-old diabetic woman was admitted to the hospital because of a sudden onset of slurred speech, weakness in both legs, and difficulty walking.

Neurologic examination revealed a left peripheral facial palsy; protrusion of the tongue to the left on extension; hypesthesia and hypalgesia of the right side of the body; dysmetria, dyssynergia, and intention tremor of the left arm; weakness in all four extremities; and bilateral Babinski signs. MRI and angiography confirmed the diagnosis.

Treatable Diseases to Be Ruled Out
Vertebral-basilar insufficiency
Vertebral aneurysm
Space-occupying lesion
Cervical spondylosis

Comment: The illustration shows the infarct in the pons involving the left facial nerve, causing the left facial palsy; the left lateral spinothalamic tract, causing the right hemihypalgesia; and the left median lemniscus, causing the right hemihypesthesia. It also shows involvement of the pyramidal tracts in the medulla, causing the quadriplegia, and the left cerebellar hemisphere, causing the dysmetria, dyssynergia, and intention tremor in the left arm. The *arrow* shows the occlusion of the basilar artery.

Synopsis: See page 125.

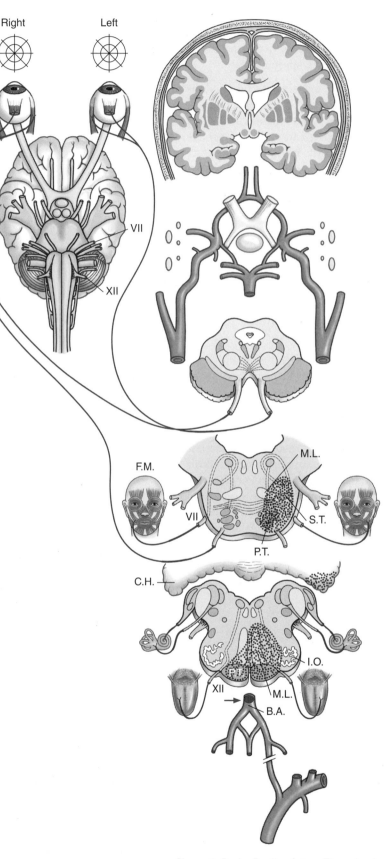

Figure 2. Brain: Basilar Artery Thrombosis

BELL'S PALSY

A 27-year-old black woman awoke one morning with "numbness" of the left side of her face, excessive tearing from her left eye, and thick speech.

Neurologic examination revealed the inability to close the left eye, Bell's phenomenon, straightening of the left nasolabial fold, and inability to retract the left side of the mouth on smiling or grimacing. Roentgenograms of the skull and mastoid were normal. An electromyogram of the left facial muscles confirmed the diagnosis.

Treatable Diseases to Be Ruled Out
Petrositis
Neurosyphilis
Cholesteatoma
Acoustic neuroma
Ramsay Hunt syndrome
Myasthenia gravis

Comment: The *arrow* in the illustration points to the damage to the left facial nerve causing paralysis of the left facial muscles.

Synopsis: In most cases, the etiology of Bell's palsy is obscure, but in some cases, reactivation of a herpes simplex virus type 1 infection or herpes zoster may be responsible. This case is typical of the way the disease presents. Diagnosis is made by electromyography and exclusion of inner ear pathology and acoustic neuroma. Bell's palsy does not cause hearing loss, so this finding should prompt further study. Treatment with corticosteroids, adrenocorticotropic hormone (ACTH; see Appendix C for details), or acyclovir may be undertaken if the patient is seen early, but it has not proven beneficial. Most cases resolve in days to months without treatment.

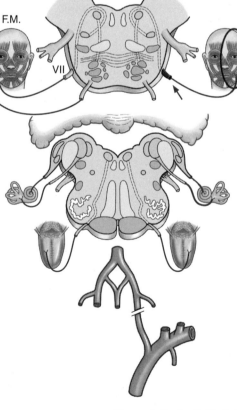

Figure 3. Brain: Bell's Palsy

BRAINSTEM GLIOMA

An 18-year-old white man complained of gradually increasing double vision for the past month. One week before he was admitted to the hospital, the right side of his mouth began to sag and his speech became dysarthric.

Neurologic examination revealed right lateral gaze palsy, right facial weakness, and hyperactive reflexes in the left extremities. Touch, pain, and vibratory sensation were diminished in the left extremities. MRI of the brain and brainstem clearly demonstrated the tumor.

Treatable Diseases to Be Ruled Out
Neurosyphilis
Tuberculous meningitis
Chordoma
Acoustic neuroma
Myasthenia gravis
Vertebral-basilar artery insufficiency

Comment: The illustration shows the tumor invading the right abducens nerve, causing right lateral gaze palsy; the right facial nerve and median lemniscus, causing loss of touch, pain, and vibratory sensation; and the pyramidal tract on the right, causing hyperactive reflexes in the right extremities.

Synopsis: Gliomas of the brainstem are unusual, but because they so closely resemble bulbar multiple sclerosis and basilar artery thrombosis, they must not be forgotten in the differential diagnosis of these conditions. Diagnosis is best made with an MRI. Treatment is usually supportive, as surgery is rarely successful. Radiation therapy may be helpful. Prognosis is poor.

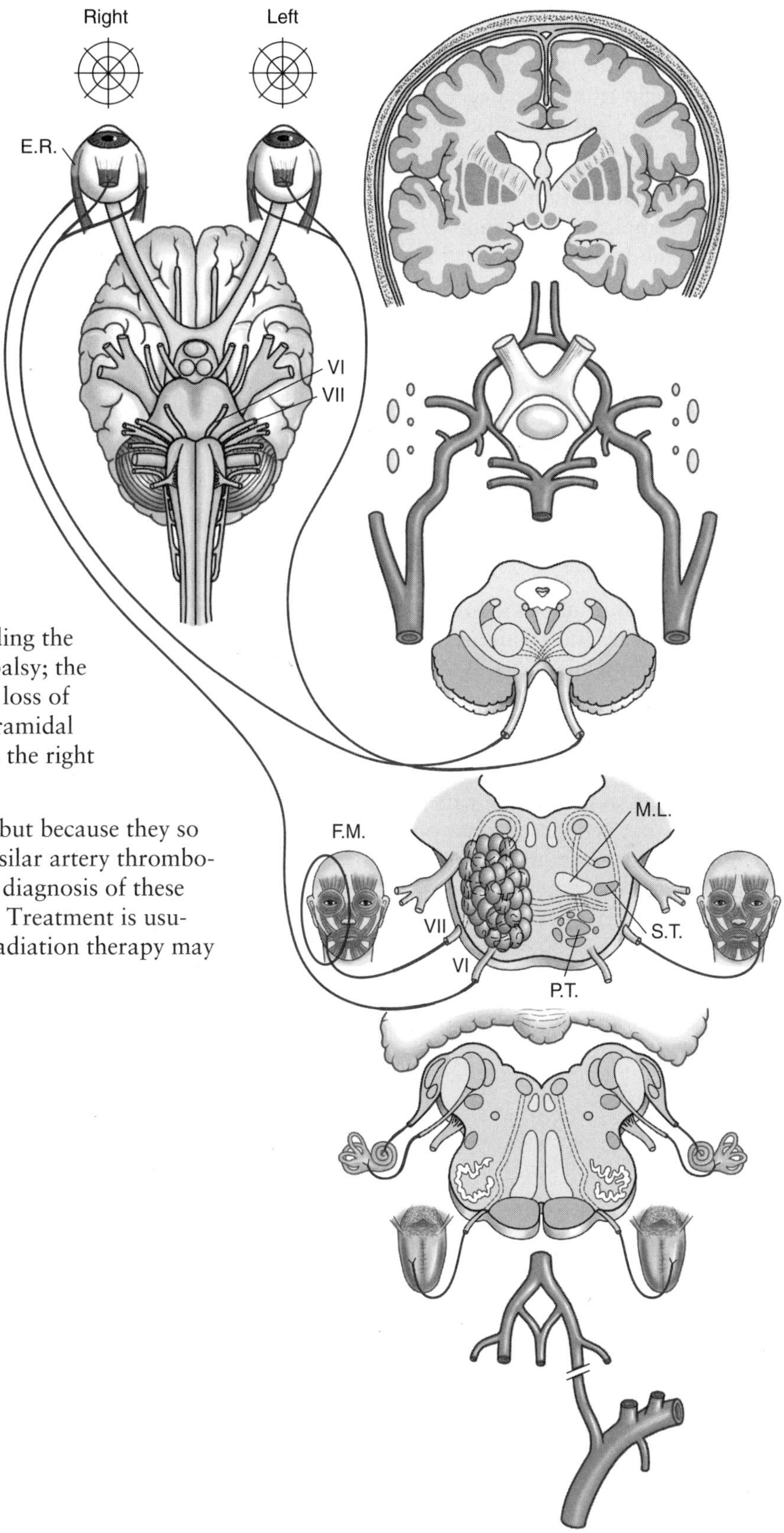

Figure 4. Brain: Brainstem Glioma

CAVERNOUS SINUS THROMBOSIS

A 38-year-old black woman with a long history of recurrent abscesses involving the right side of her nose developed sudden fever, right frontal headache, and swelling of her right eye and eyelid.

Neurologic examination revealed periorbital edema, chemosis, ptosis, exophthalmos, and complete ophthalmoplegia on the right. Funduscopic examination revealed papilledema on the right. Diagnosis was confirmed by MRI and magnetic resonance venography.

Treatable Diseases to Be Ruled Out
Wernicke's encephalopathy
Orbital cellulitis
Mucormycosis
Aneurysm of the circle of Willis
Graves' disease
Arteriovenous fistula

Comment: The thrombosis involving the right oculomotor, trochlear, and abducens nerves, causing complete right ophthalmoplegia, is illustrated.

Synopsis: Cavernous sinus thrombosis follows an extension of a bacterial infection in the paranasal sinuses, orbit, or upper half of the face into the cavernous sinus, with resulting thrombosis. Diagnosis is established by CT or MRI in most cases, but magnetic resonance venography may occasionally be necessary. Treatment with antibiotics and often anticoagulants must begin immediately if the patient is to have a chance for survival. Ultimately, the choice of antibiotic will be based on the results of blood and sinus exudate cultures.

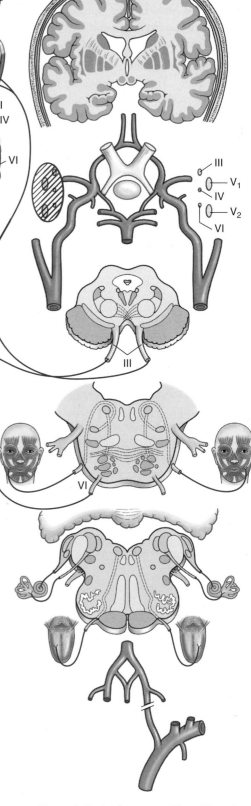

Figure 1. Brain: Cavernous Sinus Thrombosis

CEREBELLAR ABSCESS

A 12-year-old white girl developed a temperature of 103°F (39.4°C), severe pain in her right ear, and a mild yellowish aural discharge 1 week before admission to the hospital. At that time, a diagnosis of otitis media was made and the patient was treated by her primary physician. The day before admission, her fever recurred and was associated with a severe right suboccipital headache. Her mother noted that the patient staggered to the right when she walked.

Neurologic examination revealed horizontal nystagmus on right lateral gaze, a head tilt to the right, dysdiadochokinesia and dyssynergia of the right arm, and a wide-based, ataxic gait. A CT scan confirmed the diagnosis.

Treatable Diseases to Be Ruled Out
Acoustic neuroma
Cerebellar tumor
Dilantin toxicity
Meningitis

Comment: The illustration shows the involvement of the right cerebellar lobe, causing dyskinesia, nystagmus, and ataxia.

Synopsis: A cerebellar abscess usually results from an extension of an infection from the middle or inner ear, as in this case, but it may also result from hematogenous spread from the lung or heart. Organisms that cause cerebellar abscess include streptococci, staphylococci, *pseudomonas*, and anaerobes. Temporal lobe abscesses may result from the spread of infection from an otic source, whereas frontal lobe involvement is more likely to be caused by spread from the sinuses. Hematogenous spread is usually associated with multiple abscesses. Diagnosis is best made by CT or MRI. Lumbar puncture is contraindicated. The treatment of choice used to be craniotomy and surgical drainage, but needle aspiration and drainage along with systemic antibiotics may obviate the need for radical surgery. In urgent situations, intravenous penicillin (up to 20 million units per day) and metronidazole may be started while awaiting the results of culture of the drainage; otherwise, the choice of antibiotic will depend on the results of the culture.

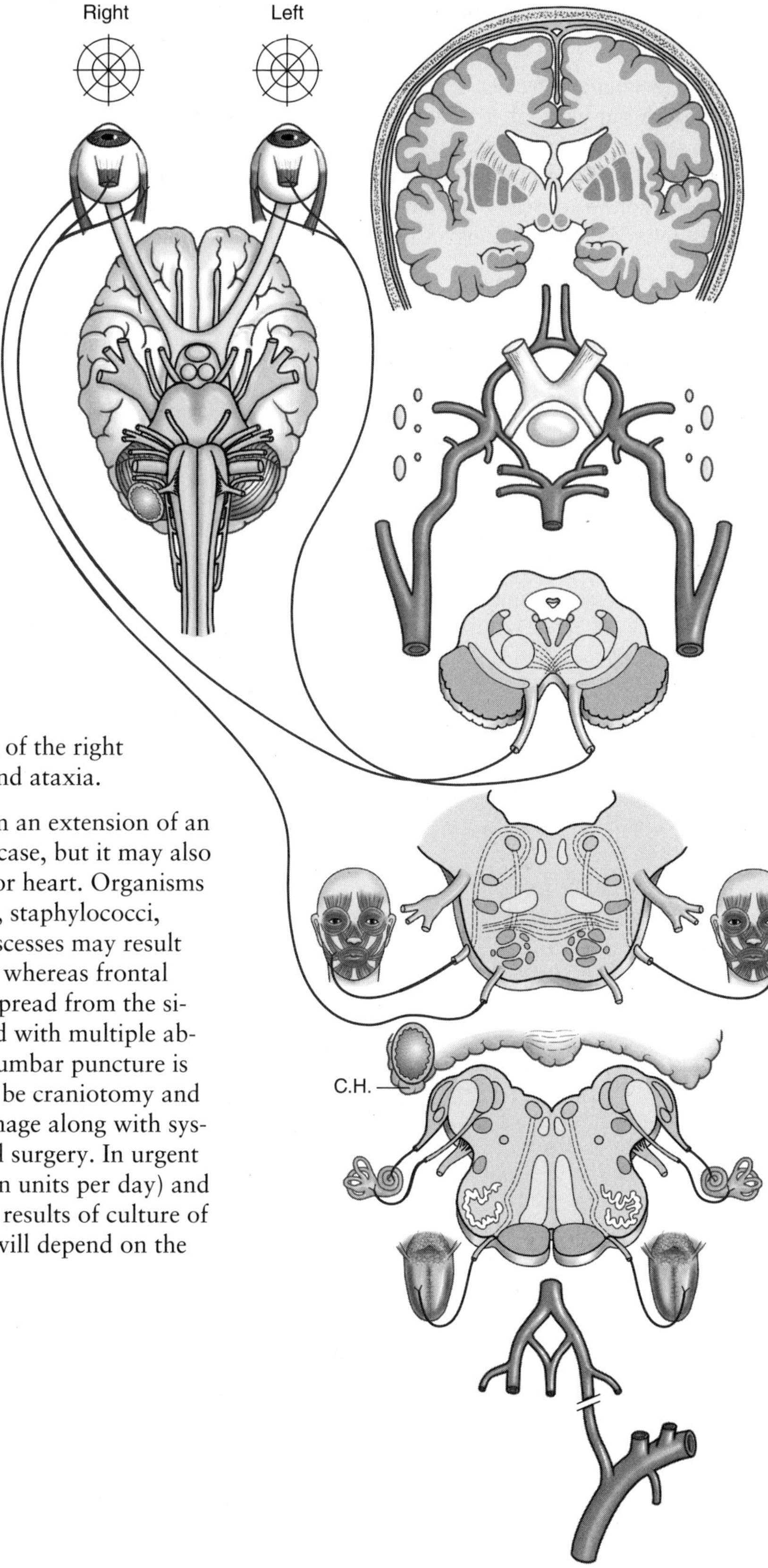

Figure 2. Brain: Cerebellar Abscess

CONVERSION HYSTERIA

A 19-year-old white man presented at the emergency department with convulsions that had been recurring for the past several days.

Neurologic examination revealed repeated episodes of clonic movements of all four extremities with forcible closing of the eyes and mouth but without significant clenching of the jaw. There were no lacerations of the tongue, incontinence, focal neurologic signs, or papilledema. Between episodes, the patient continued to keep his eyes closed and resisted efforts to open them. The examiner began a pleasant conversation with him, and after 5 minutes, the patient responded and the convulsions ceased, to everyone's surprise. The patient was referred to a psychiatrist, who found that the "convulsions" began after his parents discovered he was having an illicit affair with a young lady and threw him out of the house.

Treatable Diseases to Be Ruled Out
Space-occupying lesion of the brain
Viral encephalitis
Toxic encephalopathy
Alcohol withdrawal
Neurosyphilis
Idiopathic epilepsy

Synopsis: Hysterical convulsions are typically diagnosed by the absence of tongue lacerations and incontinence. Furthermore, there often is no tonic phase in the seizures and no postictal somnolence, as demonstrated in this case. EEG, both awake and asleep, is normal, but it is important to remember that this finding alone does not rule out epilepsy. A psychiatric consultation and psychometric testing will help confirm the diagnosis.

DILANTIN TOXICITY

A 23-year-old housewife who had epilepsy for several years complained of staggering while walking.

Neurologic examination revealed horizontal and vertical nystagmus, mild dysdiadochokinesia and dyssynergia bilaterally, and a wide-based, ataxic gait. Romberg's sign was positive but not exaggerated when the patient closed her eyes. Serum phenytoin level was 34 μg/mL. All other laboratory and radiographic studies were normal.

Treatable Diseases to Be Ruled Out
Toxic encephalopathy
Space-occupying lesion of the cerebellum

Comment: The illustration shows diffuse involvement of the cerebellum, causing nystagmus, dyskinesia, dyssynergia, and ataxia.

Synopsis: The patient in this case presented with the typical cerebellar signs of dilantin toxicity. Many other anticonvulsant drugs, such as phenobarbital, carbamazepine, and valproic acid, may cause the same clinical picture. Dilantin may also cause hypertrophic gingivitis, Hodgkin's syndrome, a "lupus" reaction, and folic acid deficiency, among other strange phenomena. Diagnosis can be confirmed by determining the serum Dilantin level, which most laboratories consider normal at the 10 to 20 μg/mL range. The treatment is to decrease or withhold the drug until the level returns to normal. Some patients have symptoms of Dilantin toxicity even though their serum levels are normal, so they must be switched to another anticonvulsant drug.

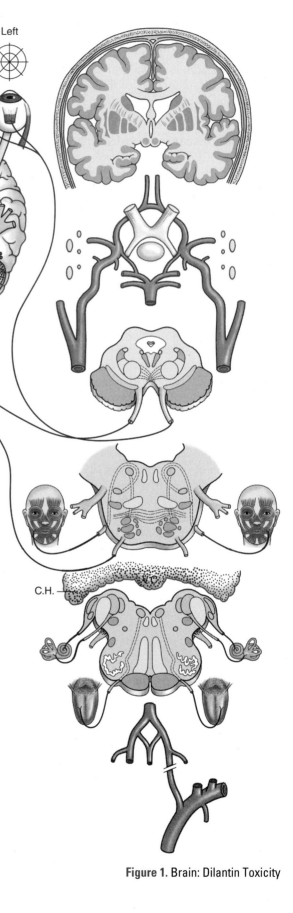

Figure 1. Brain: Dilantin Toxicity

EPIDURAL HEMATOMA

A 33-year-old white man sustained a severe blow to the head in an automobile accident and was brought to the accident ward in a semiconscious state. Shortly after admission, he was alert and cooperative. Radiography of the skull revealed a linear fracture to the right temporal bone. Within hours, the patient lapsed into a coma.

Neurologic examination revealed a blood pressure of 170/60 mm Hg; a pulse of 58 beats per minute; a dilated, areflexic right pupil; and left hemiparesis. A CT scan confirmed the diagnosis.

Treatable Diseases to Be Ruled Out
Subdural hematoma
Intracerebral hematoma
Depressed skull fracture
Toxic encephalopathy
Cerebral embolism

Comment: The illustration demonstrates the fracture (*arrow*) and the large collection of blood over the temporal-parietal area of the right hemisphere, causing the left hemiparesis. The dilated, areflexic right pupil is probably a result of uncal herniation.

Synopsis: An epidural hematoma is usually caused by a torn meningeal artery (particularly the middle meningeal artery), which leads to a rapid accumulation of blood in the epidural space and compression of the brain. Typically, the patient may be semiconscious when first seen and may have a "lucid interval" only to lapse into a coma, as in this case. Diagnosis is best made with CT. Treatment is surgical evacuation of the hematoma, although small epidural hematomas may be treated conservatively.

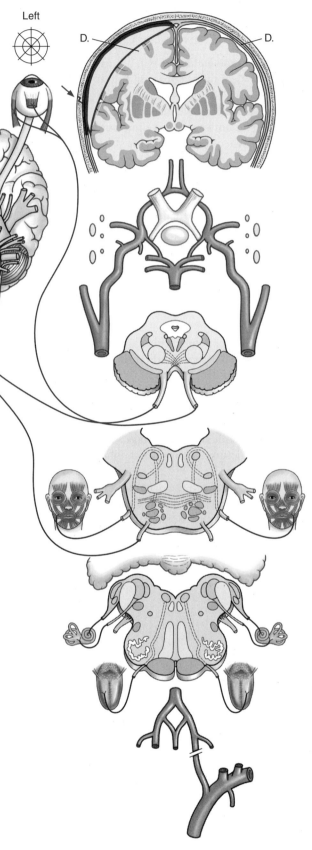

Figure 1. Brain: Epidural Hematoma

GENERAL PARESIS

A 45-year-old black man had paroxysmal attacks of severe biparietal headaches for the past 2 months. His wife stated that he had become forgetful, short-tempered, and messy in his appearance during the past year. The patient had been treated for a genital ulcer 13 years before, after several infections.

Neurologic examination revealed an inability to recall presidents or recent events, inability to interpret proverbial phrases, disorganized affect, and small, irregular pupils that did not respond to light but reacted to accommodation. A spinal fluid Venereal Disease Research Laboratory (VDRL) test was positive. A CT scan showed dilated ventricles and cortical atrophy.

Treatable Diseases to Be Ruled Out

Lead intoxication or other form of toxic encephalopathy
Space-occupying lesion of the cerebrum
Wernicke's encephalopathy

Comment: The illustration demonstrates the involvement of the leptomeninges and lining of the ventricles, as well as the diffuse cortical involvement, causing the dementia.

Synopsis: General paresis is caused by the spirochete *Treponema pallidum* invasion of the meninges and brain. The spirochetes can be demonstrated in the cortex. The incidence of primary syphilis has increased recently, especially in homosexual men, so it can be expected that the incidence of paresis will increase also. Diagnosis is by CT scan or MRI coupled with positive blood and spinal fluid serology, especially the fluorescent treponemal antibody test. Treatment is with aqueous penicillin G, doxycycline, or tetracycline, according to the dosage and administration outlined in Appendix C.

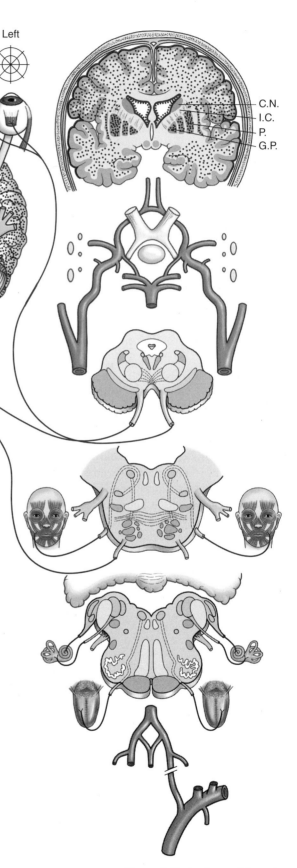

Figure 1. Brain: General Paresis

GLIOBLASTOMA MULTIFORME OF THE FRONTAL LOBE

A 46-year-old white man visited his family physician 1 week before admission to the hospital because of forgetfulness, thick speech, and right frontal headaches. One hour before admission, he became semiconscious and muttered incomprehensibly.

Neurologic examination revealed facial asymmetry, left hemiparesis, and a grasp and aftergrasp reflex of the left hand. An MRI confirmed the diagnosis.

Treatable Diseases to Be Ruled Out
General paresis
Wernicke's encephalopathy
Other space-occupying lesion of the cerebrum

Comment: The illustration shows the tumor involving the right fontal lobe, causing the stupor and right hemiparesis.

Synopsis: Glioblastoma multiforme of the frontal lobe accounts for 28% of all brain tumors and is the most malignant. Typically, this tumor presents as a cerebrovascular accident, even though the patient may have had symptoms of mild dementia for several months. Diagnosis is best established by an MRI because this imaging technique helps distinguish glioblastomas from the less-malignant astrocytomas and from other tumors that may be treated with surgery. Treatment includes surgery, radiation, and chemotherapy, but consultation with a neurosurgeon and oncologist is necessary to determine the best therapy for individual cases. Prognosis is grave for glioblastoma, but 50% or more of patients with low-grade astrocytomas survive 5 years.

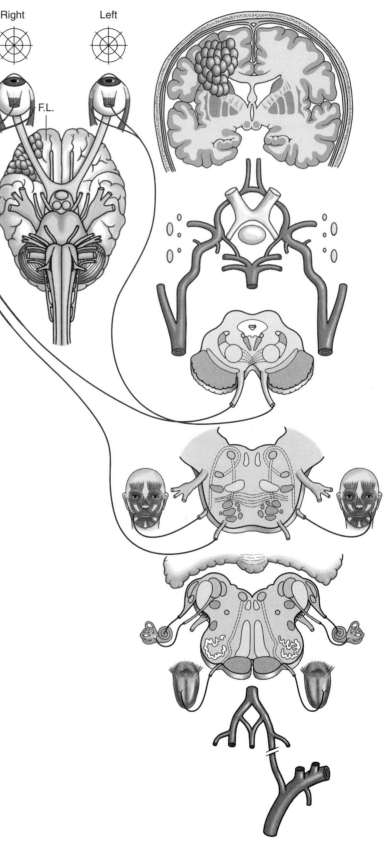

Figure 2. Brain: Glioblastoma Multiforme of the Frontal Lobe

HUNTINGTON'S CHOREA

A 39-year-old white man had involuntary lurching movements of his arms and difficulty walking for several months.

Neurologic examination disclosed choreiform movements of the arms and face; grotesque, clownish gait; slow mentation; and poor attention span. A CT scan revealed an enlarged butterfly appearance of the lateral ventricles. Genetic testing confirmed the diagnosis. The patient's father had died in a mental institution at the age of 45.

Treatable Diseases to Be Ruled Out
Phenothiazine intoxication
Wilson's disease
Manganese toxicity

Comment: The illustration demonstrates the diffuse involvement of the cerebral cortex, basal ganglia, and caudate nuclei.

Synopsis: Huntington's chorea is an autosomal dominant disorder that results from a mutation of the Huntington gene on chromosome 4p1.3. Clinically, the patient first develops moodiness, antisocial behavior, and emotional lability, then as the disease progresses, cognitive difficulties and chorea. A few patients may present with the typical parkinsonian picture of rigidity and akinesia. Diagnosis can be established by genetic testing. Treatment is symptomatic; haloperidol (0.5 to 4 mg four times a day) may control the chorea. Patients may survive 11 to 30 years after diagnosis; death is usually the result of pulmonary complications or trauma.

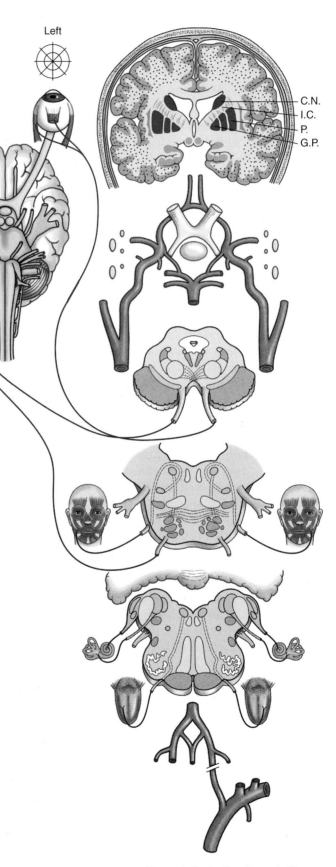

Figure 1. Brain: Huntington's Chorea

INTERNAL CAROTID ANEURYSM

A 54-year-old black homemaker noted sudden sharp, throbbing, severe pain over her left eyebrow. One hour later, she was unable to open her left eye. She was admitted to the hospital the next day.

Neurologic examination revealed a left ptosis; paralysis of upward, downward, and medial gaze; a dilated, areflexic pupil; and loss of the left corneal reflex. A left carotid angiogram confirmed the diagnosis.

Treatable Diseases to Be Ruled Out
Neurosyphilis
Tuberculous meningitis
Orbital cellulitis
Wernicke's encephalopathy
Cavernous sinus thrombosis
Sphenoid ridge meningioma
Myasthenia gravis

Comment: The illustration shows the aneurysm compressing the oculomotor nerve, causing internal and external ophthalmoplegia and ptosis, and the trigeminal nerve, causing the loss of the corneal reflex.

Synopsis: This case illustrates a frequent presentation of an unruptured cerebral aneurysm. Saccular aneurysms are congenital and typically occur at the bifurcation of the arteries in the circle of Willis, particularly the internal carotid with the posterior communicating artery. They may occur in the vertebral-basilar artery circulation as well, in which case they can mimic acoustic neuromas in symptomatology. Other aneurysm types include mycotic aneurysms associated with bacterial endocarditis, which are prone to rupture, and fusiform aneurysms due to arteriosclerosis, which are less likely to rupture. Diagnosis is best made with cerebral angiography; a four-vessel study should be done, as multiple aneurysms often occur. MRI and CT may help diagnose an aneurysm, particularly if there is rupture and subarachnoid hemorrhage. Treatment of a saccular aneurysm is surgical, and the outcome is good when the newer microsurgical technique is performed. Immediate consultation with a neurosurgeon is essential. He or she will decide whether a procedure is indicated as well as the best type of procedure for the individual case.

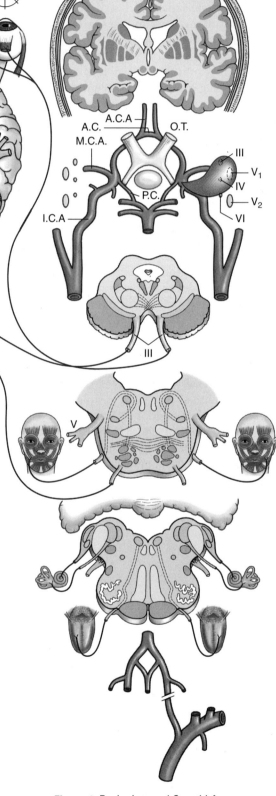

Figure 1. Brain: Internal Carotid Aneurysm

INTRACEREBRAL HEMORRHAGE

A 49-year-old hypertensive man had a severe bifrontal headache as he was returning home from work one evening. His wife noted that he was confused and went straight to bed. One hour later, she was unable to rouse him.

Neurologic examination revealed a comatose patient breathing deeply, with dilated, fixed pupils. There was little spontaneous movement of the left extremities; the right extremities failed to move, even when supraorbital pressure was applied. A CT scan confirmed the diagnosis.

Treatable Diseases to Be Ruled Out
Ruptured intracranial aneurysm
Cerebral embolism
Arteriovenous anomaly
Blood dyscrasia
Toxic encephalopathy
Diabetic coma
Meningitis

Comment: The illustration shows the hemorrhage involving the internal capsule on the left.

Synopsis: Most cases of intracerebral hemorrhage are the result of long-standing hypertension that causes weakening of the walls of the arterioles and subsequent rupture. Other causes include amyloid angiopathy of the elderly, blood dyscrasia, illicit drug use, arteriovenous malformations, and excessive anticoagulation. Diagnosis is best established by CT because it demonstrates bleeding better than MRI. Treatment consists of aggressive measures to reduce intracranial pressure (see Appendix C), including, in some cases, surgical evacuation of the blood clot. Nevertheless, prognosis is poor, with a mortality rate of almost 50%.

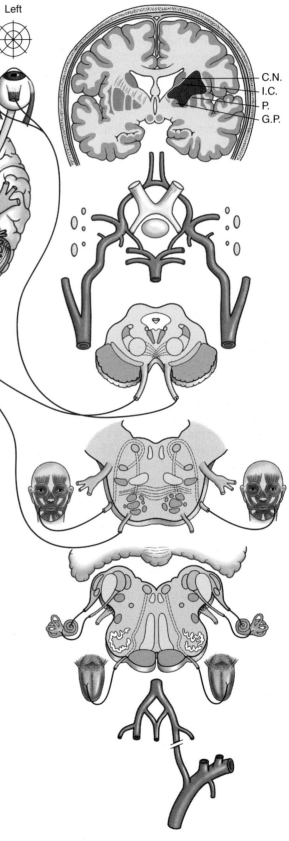

Right   Left

C.N.
I.C.
P.
G.P.

Figure 2. Brain: Intracerebral Hemorrhage

LACUNAR INFARCTION

A 73-year-old hypertensive woman complained of weakness in her left arm and leg.

Neurologic examination revealed a left-central facial palsy, deviation of the tongue to the left, weakness of the left extremities, and a left Babinski sign. MRI demonstrated an infarction of the right internal capsule.

Treatable Diseases to Be Ruled Out
Subdural hematoma
Cerebral abscess
Cerebral aneurysm
Carotid artery stenosis
Neurosyphilis
Cerebral embolism

Comment: Illustrated here is the infarction of the right internal capsule causing the left-central facial palsy and hemiparesis.

Synopsis: Lacunar infarctions are caused by the occlusion of the small penetrating branches of the middle cerebral or basilar artery supplying the internal capsule or pons. The stroke may be pure motor or pure sensory. Another clinical presentation is dysarthria with clumsy hand syndrome. Lacunar infarcts seem to be associated with hypertension (as in this case), diabetes mellitus, heavy alcohol consumption, and smoking. Diagnosis is best established by CT or MRI. It is important to rule out an embolic source with a carotid duplex scan, ECG, and echocardiography. Treatment is usually supportive because anticoagulants and antiplatelet agents (e.g., aspirin) are either contraindicated because of hypertension or have proven to be of little value.

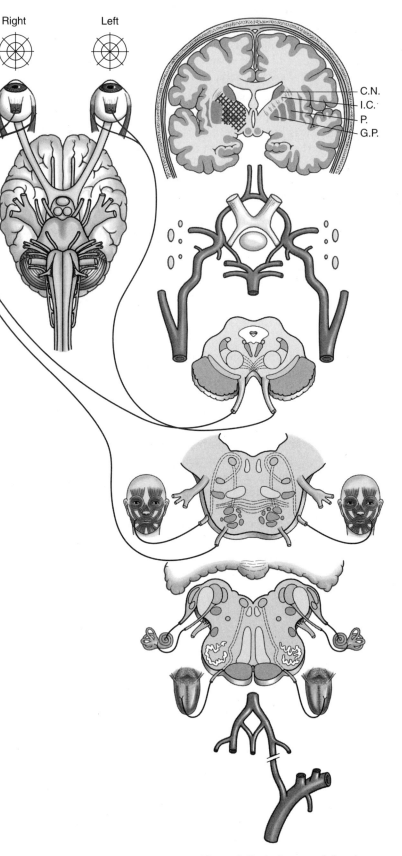

Right   Left

C.N.
I.C.
P.
G.P.

Figure 1. Brain: Lacunar Infarction

MALINGERING

A 34-year-old store clerk complained of severe low back pain radiating down her left leg since she fell on a slippery floor at work. She denied any previous history of back pain. She recently had filed a workers' compensation claim.

Neurologic examination revealed diffuse hypesthesia and hypalgesia, which did not follow a dermatomal distribution, in the left leg. The patient walked with a consistent limp favoring her left leg. Straight leg–raising test was positive on the left, regardless of whether the leg was flexed or extended at the knee. Reflexes were symmetric and active in all four extremities, and there were no other positive neurologic findings. Laboratory and radiographic studies were normal. A private investigator videotaped the patient carrying bags of groceries to her car at a supermarket with no apparent limp or other difficulties.

Treatable Diseases to Be Ruled Out
Herniated lumbar disc
Compression fracture of the spine
Sciatic neuritis
Cauda equina tumor

Synopsis: This case demonstrates the typical presentation of malingering. There is always secondary gain (usually financial, as in this case), but it may not be apparent. Nondermatomal sensory loss and a positive straight leg–raising test are common findings. Despite the limp favoring one leg, there is usually no appreciable atrophy. The only "cure" for a case such as this is a big settlement.

MEDULLOBLASTOMA

A 9-year-old boy had double vision, headaches, and a staggering gait for 2 weeks before admission to the hospital. Shortly before admission, his headaches became more severe and were associated with nausea and vomiting.

Neurologic examination revealed papilledema, paralysis of lateral gaze bilaterally, tilting of the head to the left, and wide-based truncal ataxia. A CT scan confirmed the diagnosis.

Treatable Diseases to Be Ruled Out
Dilantin toxicity
Cerebellar abscess
Meningitis
Subdural hematoma
Cysticercosis of the fourth ventricle
Subarachnoid hemorrhage

Comment: The illustration shows the tumor invading the cerebellar vermis, causing the ataxia, and compressing the fourth ventricle, causing the papilledema, headaches, and vomiting.

Synopsis: This case is typical of the way patients with medulloblastoma present. This tumor is congenital, and a specific chromosomal abnormality is found in 33% of cases. Diagnosis is best established with MRI. Neurosurgical treatment has been successful in most cases. Chemotherapy is also useful; however, an oncologist should always be consulted. The overall 5-year survival rate is at least 50%.

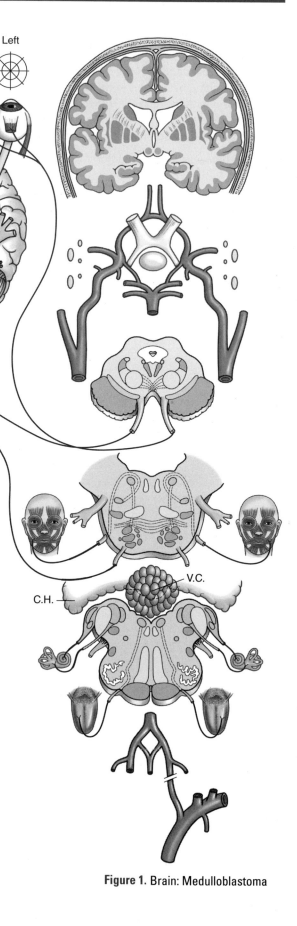

Figure 1. Brain: Medulloblastoma

MENIERE'S DISEASE

A 45-year-old white man had episodes of vertigo, tinnitus, and fullness in his left ear for the past 3 years. He had also noticed progressive loss of hearing for some time, and his hearing was further diminished in his left ear during the attacks of vertigo.

Neurologic examination during an attack revealed nystagmus on left lateral gaze; left perceptive deafness, especially to low tones; and a positive Romberg test. Electronystagmography revealed a hypoactive left labyrinth. CT and spinal fluid examination were normal. Audiograms showed perceptive deafness bilaterally, worse on the left with recruitment.

Treatable Diseases to Be Ruled Out

Neurosyphilis
Petrositis
Acoustic neuroma
Cholesteatoma
Vertebral-basilar insufficiency
Migraine
Epilepsy

Comment: The illustration shows the involvement of the labyrinths and cochlea bilaterally but worse on the left, causing vertigo, tinnitus, and deafness.

Synopsis: The etiology of Meniere's disease is unclear, but a few cases may be hereditary. The mechanism for the attacks seems to be swelling of the endolymphatic system for unknown reasons. Diagnosis is primarily by exclusion of serious conditions with CT or MRI. Medical treatment with antihistamines and anticholinergics is beneficial in most cases. Diuretics have also been used. When the condition is disabling, surgical procedures are indicated (see Appendix C).

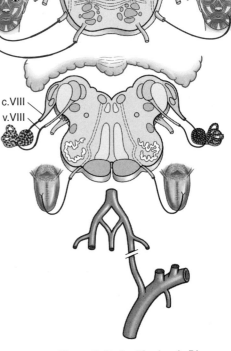

Figure 2. Brain: Meniere's Disease

METASTATIC CARCINOMA

A 56-year-old white man had a sudden jacksonian convulsion that began in his left leg. He was admitted to the hospital in a stuporous state. His wife stated that he was a heavy smoker for many years and suffered from a chronic cigarette cough. Occasionally, he coughed up small amounts of blood.

Neurologic examination on admission revealed flaccid paralysis of the left leg and, to a lesser extent, the left arm, and a left Babinski sign. Neurologic examination the following morning revealed impaired judgment and loss of memory of recent events. A CT scan clearly demonstrated the two lesions in the cerebral cortex. Chest radiography and bronchoscopy confirmed the diagnosis of bronchogenic carcinoma.

Treatable Diseases to Be Ruled Out
Space-occupying lesion
Transient ischemic attack
Cerebral emboli

Comment: The illustration demonstrates a large metastasis to the right parasagittal area, causing the paralysis of the left leg, and a smaller metastasis to the temporal lobe, causing the impaired judgment and memory loss.

Synopsis: Cerebral metastasis occurs from a large variety of neoplasms, especially from the breast, lung, and pelvis. Diagnosis is best established by MRI with contrast coupled with a search for the primary neoplasm. If only one or two lesions are present, treatment is surgical. When multiple lesions are observed, radiotherapy and chemotherapy may be useful in improving mortality and morbidity. A neurosurgeon and oncologist should be consulted for management.

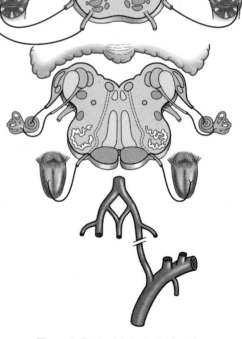

Figure 3. Brain: Metastatic Carcinoma

MIDDLE CEREBRAL ARTERY THROMBOSIS

A 62-year-old white man noted a mild biparietal headache and slight weakness in his right arm and hand when he went to bed one evening. The following morning, his wife found him unable to speak or to move his right arm or leg.

Neurologic examination revealed expressive aphasia but normal comprehension, right central palsy, right hemiparesis (more marked in the arm than the leg), a mild loss of position and vibratory senses on the right, and astereognosis in the right hand. Angiography revealed a 90% stenosis of the left carotid artery at the bifurcation, and occlusion of the left middle cerebral artery.

Treatable Diseases to Be Ruled Out
Subdural hematoma
Carotid artery stenosis or plaque
Brain abscess
Neurosyphilis
Cerebral embolism
Collagen disease
Blood dyscrasia

Comment: The illustration shows the infarction in the left middle cerebral artery distribution, causing the weakness and sensory changes in the right extremities and the expressive aphasia, and the occlusion of the left middle cerebral artery (*arrow*).

Synopsis: See page 125.

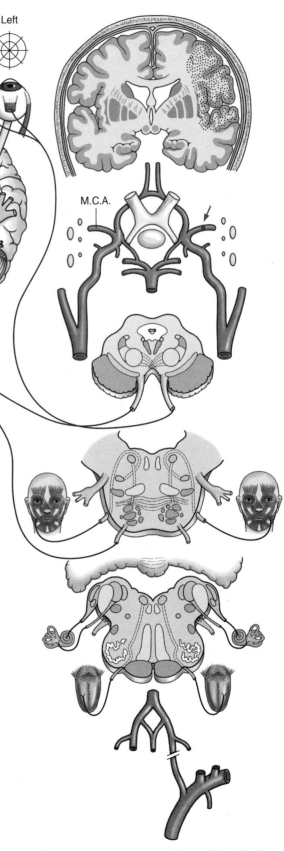

Figure 4. Brain: Middle Cerebral Artery Thrombosis

MULTIPLE SCLEROSIS (BULBAR)

A 29-year-old white man had intermittent staggering gait, dizziness, and double vision for the past year. One week before admission to the hospital, he developed a blind spot in his left visual field.

Neurologic examination revealed a left paracentral scotoma, disconjugate lateral gaze, perceptive deafness on the left, dysdiadochokinesia, and an intention tremor in the left upper extremity. The patient also had a wide-based ataxic gait and hyperactive reflexes in the right extremities. An MRI showed multiple plaques throughout the brain and brainstem. Spinal fluid examination revealed an elevated myelin basic protein level.

Treatable Diseases to Be Ruled Out
Neurosyphilis
Cerebellar abscess
Acoustic neuroma
Vertebral artery aneurysm
Vertebral-basilar insufficiency
Platybasia

Comment: The illustration demonstrates the involvement of the optic nerve, causing the paracentral scotoma; the median longitudinal fasciculus, causing the disconjugate gaze; the restiform body, causing the ataxia and dyskinesia; and the pyramidal tract, causing the hyperactive reflexes in the right extremities.

Synopsis: See page 102.

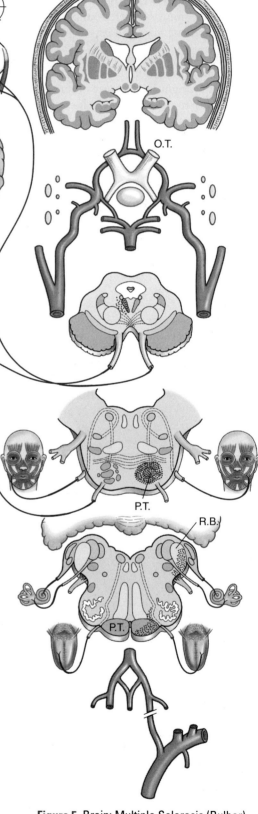

Figure 5. Brain: Multiple Sclerosis (Bulbar)

MYASTHENIA GRAVIS

A 26-year-old white woman complained of intermittent double vision that occurred most often toward the end of the day. She switched eyeglasses several times, but there was no improvement in her vision. One week before admission to the hospital, she had an upper respiratory infection. Two days after the onset of the infection, she developed ptosis of her left eyelid.

Neurologic examination revealed left ptosis; partial paralysis of left upward, medial, and downward gaze; and total paralysis of right lateral gaze. There was complete remission of symptoms and signs after intravenous administration of edrophonium (0.5 mL [Tensilon; ICN Pharmaceuticals, Costa Mesa, CA]).

Treatable Diseases to Be Ruled Out
Neurosyphilis
Tuberculous meningitis
Wernicke's encephalopathy
Sphenoid ridge meningioma
Aneurysm of the circle of Willis
Hyperthyroidism

Comment: The illustration shows the involvement of the left oculomotor myoneural junctions (*arrows*), causing the left ptosis and paresis of left upward, medial, and downward gaze, and the right abducens myoneural junction (*arrow*), causing the right lateral gaze palsy.

Synopsis: Myasthenia gravis is an autoimmune disease in which antibodies attack the acetylcholine receptor sites at the myoneural junctions, causing ocular muscle involvement, as in this case, dysphagia, dysarthria, and, less commonly, weakness in the extremities. Another rare condition, called *Lambert-Eaton myasthenic syndrome*, may also affect the myoneural junctions but more often involves the extremities and respiratory muscles and is often associated with small cell carcinoma of the lung. The diagnosis of myasthenia gravis is made by the Tensilon test, as in this case, or the finding of acetylcholine receptor antibodies, as in 60% to 90% of cases. Patients without acetylcholine receptor antibodies may have antibodies against other muscle surface proteins, such as muscle-specific tyrosine kinase. Elderly patients should have a CT scan of the chest to rule out a thymoma. Treatment is with acetylcholinesterase inhibitors such as pyridostigmine (Mestinon; Valeant Pharmaceuticals, Costa Mesa, CA), corticosteroids, and immunosuppressant drugs (see Appendix C). Plasmapheresis is useful for myasthenic crisis, but the results are short term. Thymectomy is often recommended for everyone except patients with ocular myasthenia. Prognosis is good in most cases, but a few patients die from respiratory failure or pneumonia.

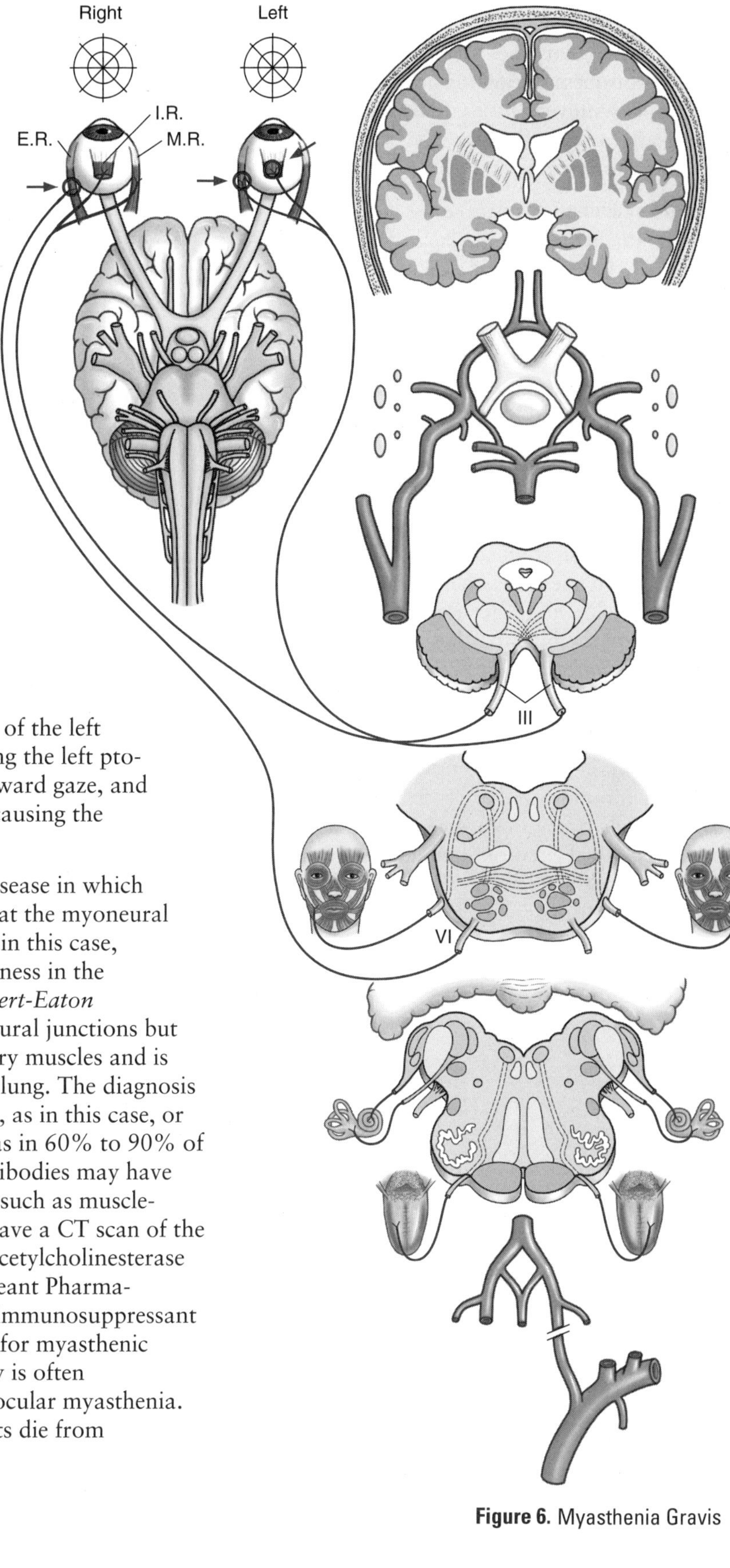

Figure 6. Myasthenia Gravis

OLFACTORY GROOVE MENINGIOMA

A 52-year-old white man complained of unrelenting frontal headache of 1 year's duration. His family noted that he evinced very little interest in his business during the past year, and he responded with very little emotion to the sudden death of his wife, 6 months before he was admitted to the hospital.

Neurologic examination revealed left-sided anosmia, optic atrophy, and concentric narrowing of the left visual field. The patient also had papilledema of the right disc and considerable loss of memory of recent events. A CT scan confirmed the diagnosis.

Treatable Diseases to Be Ruled Out
General paresis
Toxic encephalopathy
Other space-occupying lesion
Normal pressure hydrocephalus

Comment: The illustration shows the tumor compressing the optic nerve, causing concentric narrowing of the visual field and Foster Kennedy syndrome, and the pressure on the olfactory bulb, causing the anosmia. (Foster Kennedy syndrome is homolateral optic atrophy and contralateral papilledema.)

Synopsis: Meningiomas are benign tumors originating in the meninges in many locations in the brain. They account for 20% to 30% of brain tumors and are twice as frequent in women. Diagnosis can be made by radiography of the skull, CT, or MRI. Treatment with surgical excision is curative in most cases, although recurrences are not uncommon. Radiation and chemotherapy may be necessary for treating recurrent meningiomas.

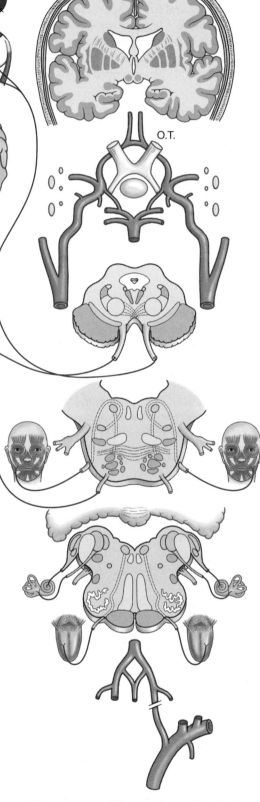

Figure 1. Brain: Olfactory Groove Meningioma

PARASAGITTAL MENINGIOMA

A 39-year-old white woman had a 3-year history of left-sided jacksonian convulsions beginning in her left leg. One year before admission to the hospital, she developed weakness in her left leg and intermittent right frontal headache.

Neurologic examination revealed marked weakness of extension and flexion of the left foot and toes, hyperactive and pathologic reflexes of the left leg and foot, and hyperostosis of the skull in the right parasagittal area.

Comment: The illustration shows the involvement of the right parasagittal area, causing weakness and hyperactive reflexes in the left leg and foot.

Synopsis: The parasagittal area is another common place for meningiomas to develop. Diagnosis can be made by CT or MRI, but the neurosurgeon may prefer an MRI or magnetic resonance angiography to determine the extent of the involvement of the superior sagittal sinus. The clinician should consider the possibility of a parasagittal meningioma in patients who present with isolated weakness in the lower extremities, even though this symptom is more likely to be related to a tumor involving the spinal cord or nerve roots.

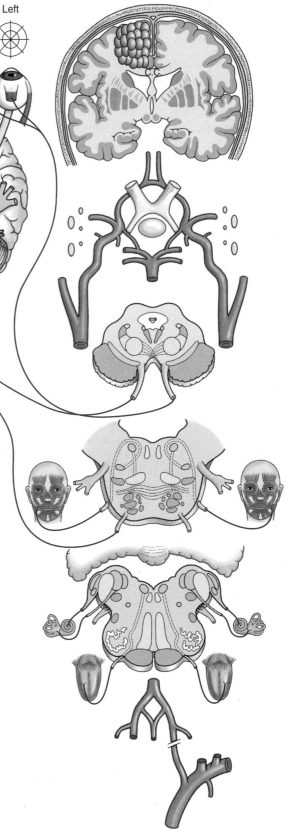

Right   Left

Figure 1. Brain: Parasagittal Meningioma

PARKINSON'S DISEASE

A 50-year-old nurse has had a tremor in her right hand and difficulty in writing legibly for the past 2 months.

Neurologic examination revealed masked facies and a mild tremor of the right hand and, to a lesser extent, the left hand; the tremors were more noticeable when the patient was at rest. The patient also had a short-stepped gait and a stooped posture. Diagnostic studies were unremarkable.

Treatable Diseases to Be Ruled Out
Wilson's disease
Phenothiazine intoxication
Hyperthyroidism
Manganese toxicity

Comment: The illustration shows the asymmetric involvement of the basal ganglia and substantia nigra responsible for the tremor, rigidity, and gait disturbances.

Synopsis: Most cases of Parkinson's disease are idiopathic, but a few are hereditary, especially if it develops in the third or fourth decade, or postencephalitic. The diagnosis is made on the basis of the clinical picture and the exclusion of other disorders that may cause tremor and gait disturbances. Treatment usually begins with a combination of levodopa and carbidopa, such as Sinemet (Merck & Co., West Point, PA). Later, a dopamine agonist such as pergolide or pramipexole is added. Selegiline has not proven effective in delaying the progression of the disease. Dosages and schedules for these drugs are outlined in Appendix C. Recently, interest in pallidotomy has returned, and deep brain stimulation has proven beneficial. A neurosurgeon should be consulted. Physiotherapy should be started early.

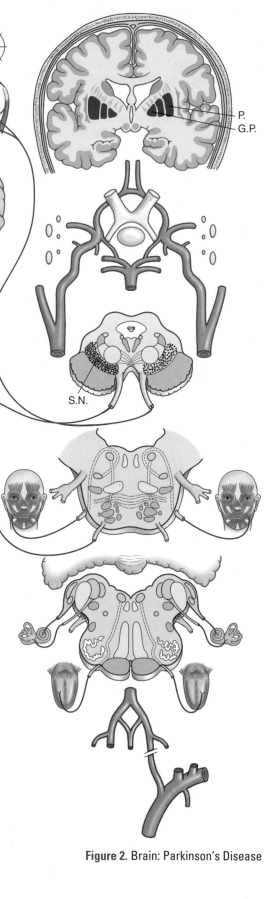

Figure 2. Brain: Parkinson's Disease

PINEALOMA

A 7-year-old white boy was examined because he developed pubic hair and an enlarged penis during the past 4 months. He also experienced intermittent headaches.

Neurologic examination revealed bilateral upward gaze palsy (Parinaud's syndrome), questionable paresis of convergence, and bilateral papilledema. A CT scan confirmed the diagnosis.

Treatable Diseases to Be Ruled Out
Wernicke's encephalopathy
Myasthenia gravis
Hyperthyroidism

Comment: The illustration shows the tumor in the aqueduct of Sylvius compressing the oculomotor nerves and neighboring structures (*arrow*), causing paralysis of upward gaze and convergence. The obstruction of the aqueduct leads to hydrocephalus and papilledema. Pinealomas rarely secrete the gonadotropic hormones that cause precocious puberty, as in this case.

Synopsis: Pineal tumors are rare and may originate in germ, pineal, or glial cells. Occasionally, a meningioma or pineal cyst occurs in this region. Headache is the most common presenting symptom. Diagnosis is best made by MRI. All patients must be treated surgically, but radiation and chemotherapy may be needed as well for malignant tumors, once a histologic diagnosis is established. Prognosis is good in most cases.

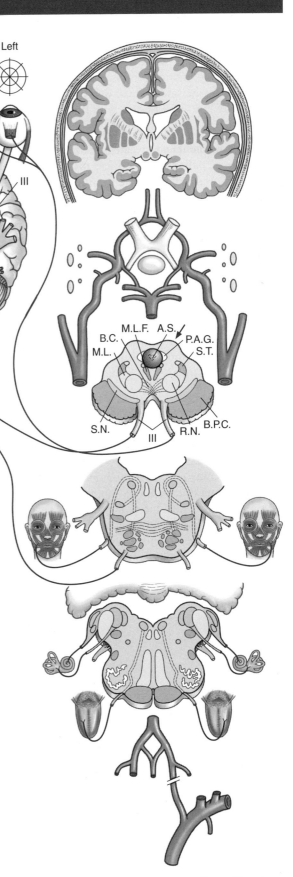

Figure 3. Brain: Pinealoma

PITUITARY ADENOMA

A 45-year-old white woman had failing vision in both eyes for the past 2 years that was not improved by changing eyeglass prescriptions several times. She said that during the past 6 months, she felt "like a horse with blinders on."

Neurologic examination revealed bitemporal hemianopsia, pallor of both discs, and loss of axillary and pubic hair. A roentgenogram of the skull revealed ballooning of the sella turcica. A CT scan confirmed the diagnosis.

Treatable Diseases to Be Ruled Out
Neurosyphilis
Craniopharyngioma
Tuberculum sellae meningioma
Aneurysm of the circle of Willis

Comment: The illustration shows the tumor compressing the optic chiasm, causing the bitemporal hemianopsia, and the pituitary gland, causing the loss of axillary and pubic hair due to hypopituitarism.

Synopsis: Pituitary adenomas may be very small (microadenomas) or may be 1 cm or larger. They may invade the hypothalamus, causing diabetes insipidus, or compress the third, fourth, and sixth cranial nerves, causing ophthalmoplegia. Rarely, they may compress the brainstem, causing papilledema. If the adenoma is a secreting tumor, the patient may present with Cushing's syndrome or acromegaly. Diagnosis is best established by MRI, which is successful in detecting even microadenomas. Treatment includes hormone replacement and surgical excision using the transsphenoidal approach, followed by radiation if necessary. A neurosurgeon can best determine the approach to treatment in each case. Prognosis is good, but recurrences are not infrequent.

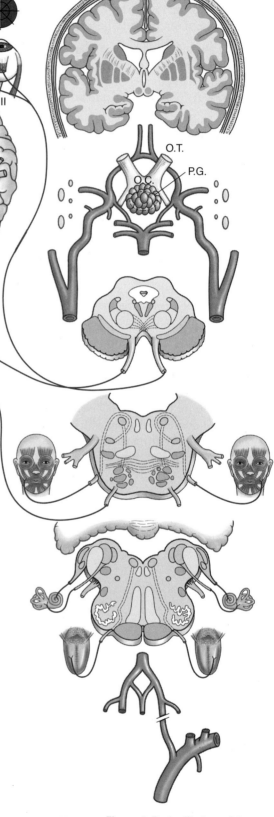

Figure 4. Brain: Pituitary Adenoma

POSTERIOR CEREBRAL ARTERY EMBOLISM

A 28-year-old white woman with a known history of rheumatic valvulitis and atrial fibrillation experienced sudden blindness in the left half of her visual field and an occipital headache.

Neurologic examination revealed a left homonymous hemianopsia with macular sparing. A CT scan demonstrated the infarction of the right occipital and temporal lobes.

Treatable Diseases to Be Ruled Out
Space-occupying lesion of the cerebrum
Arteriovenous anomaly
Subacute bacterial endocarditis
Collagen disease
Blood dyscrasia
Vertebral-basilar insufficiency
Neurosyphilis

Comment: The illustration shows the infarction of the right occipital lobe, causing left homonymous hemianopsia with macular sparing. The *arrow* points to the occlusion of the left posterior cerebral artery.

Synopsis: A cerebral embolism, in contrast to cerebral thrombosis, is almost always sudden in onset. The resulting infarct is usually ischemic but may be hemorrhagic, which makes the diagnosis and treatment difficult. Diagnosis is best established by the findings of an infarction on CT or MRI and by locating the embolism's source. Cerebral emboli most commonly originate from a mural thrombus following myocardial infarction; a thrombus in the atrium due to chronic atrial fibrillation, as in this case; subacute or acute bacterial endocarditis; or an atherosclerotic plaque in the aorta or a carotid or vertebral artery. Other causes are atrial myxoma, cardiomyopathies, and paradoxical, fat, and air embolisms. Treatment of most cerebral emboli is anticoagulation with heparin first, followed by warfarin sodium in the outpatient department. Stroke rehabilitation should begin immediately.

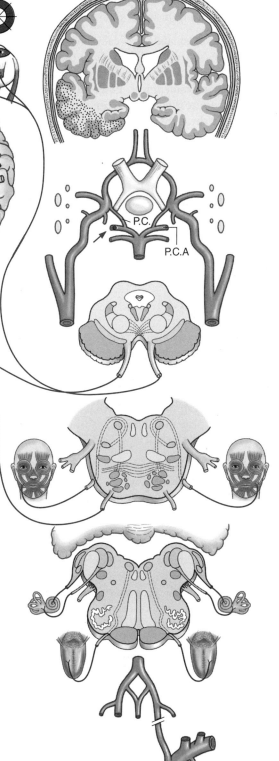

Figure 5. Brain: Posterior Cerebral Artery Embolism

POSTERIOR INFERIOR CEREBELLAR ARTERY THROMBOSIS

A 58-year-old businessman suddenly developed a high-pitched ringing in his right ear, dizziness, and right facial pain.

Neurologic examination revealed nystagmus on right lateral gaze, partial ptosis of the right eyelid, constriction of the right pupil, and right perceptive deafness. Finger-to-nose and heel-to-knee testing revealed an intention tremor on the right. In addition, there was loss of sensation to pain and temperature on the right side of the face and the left trunk and extremities, and a positive Romberg test. MRI of the brain and brainstem revealed the infarction of the medulla, and four-vessel angiography demonstrated the occlusion of the posterior inferior cerebral artery.

Treatable Diseases to Be Ruled Out
Cerebellar abscess
Acoustic neuroma
Vertebral aneurysm
Meniere's disease
Vertebral-basilar insufficiency

Comment: The illustration shows the infarction in the right lateral medulla involving the restiform body, causing the intention tremor and the patient's falling to the right on Romberg's test; lateral spinothalamic tract and descending tract of the trigeminal nerve, causing crossed hemianalgesia; and the vestibular nucleus, causing nystagmus.

Synopsis: See page 125 for a discussion of the etiology, treatment, and differential diagnoses of cerebral thrombosis, including cerebellar abscess, acoustic neuroma, vertebral aneurysm, Meniere's disease, multiple sclerosis, and vertebral-basilar insufficiency. Cerebral abscess can be excluded because it has a more insidious onset, with fever and probable middle ear infection or infection with another bacterium. Acoustic neuroma and vertebral aneurysm have the same symptoms as posterior inferior cerebellar artery thrombosis, but they have a slowly progressive onset and are often associated with headache. Meniere's disease is not associated with long tract signs or facial pain. Multiple sclerosis is not likely to present with all these symptoms at once; moreover, it is characterized by exacerbations and remissions. Vertebral-basilar artery insufficiency is associated with multiple transient ischemic attacks, and neurologic examinations between attacks are often normal.

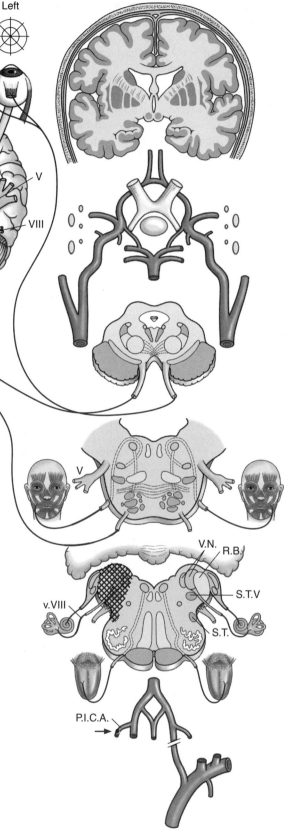

Figure 6. Brain: Posterior Inferior Cerebellar Artery Thrombosis

ST. LOUIS ENCEPHALITIS

A 23-year-old black man developed a severe occipital headache, nausea, vomiting, and drowsiness just before he was admitted to the hospital.

Neurologic examination revealed the patient to be semiconscious, uncontrollable, and irrational. He moved all four extremities but exhibited bilateral Babinski signs. His temperature was 102°F (38.8°C). Spinal fluid examination revealed an opening pressure of 350 mm H_2O, 135 white blood cells/mm^3 (predominantly lymphocytes), and normal glucose and chloride levels. That evening, the patient lapsed into a coma and never regained consciousness.

Treatable Diseases to Be Ruled Out
Toxic encephalopathy
Diabetic coma
Insulin shock
Wernicke's encephalopathy
Lead encephalopathy
Bacterial meningitis
Space-occupying lesion of the cerebrum

Comment: The illustration reveals the diffuse involvement of the cerebral cortex and meninges; however, the thalamus and midbrain are more involved, leading to the delirium and coma.

Synopsis: St. Louis encephalitis is caused by a mosquito-transmitted flavivirus. It usually occurs in the summer and fall. Viral encephalitis may be caused by a host of viruses, including enteroviruses, togaviruses, retroviruses, adenoviruses, and herpesviruses. Diagnosis is usually made by isolating the virus from the blood, spinal fluid, or tissue, or with animal inoculation, serologic tests, and amplification of viral nucleic acids. Treatment is now available for several viruses, including acyclovir for herpes simplex virus, ganciclovir and foscarnet for cytomegalovirus, reverse transcriptase and protease inhibitors for human immunodeficiency virus, and famciclovir for varicella-zoster virus. The reader is referred to standard infectious disease texts for definite treatment schedules. The prognosis is good in most cases of St. Louis encephalitis, but the mortality rate may reach 20%.

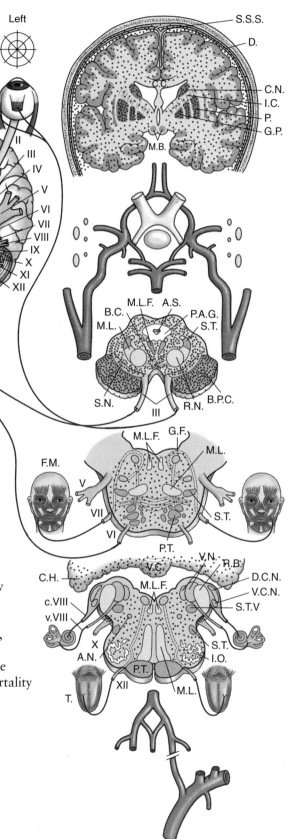

Figure 1. Brain: St. Louis Encephalitis

SUBARACHNOID HEMORRHAGE

A 36-year-old homemaker developed a sudden acute generalized headache, nausea, and vomiting. By the time she reached the emergency department, she was in a semiconscious state.

Neurologic examination revealed subhyaloid hemorrhages of the retina, dilated pupils, roving extraocular movements, nuchal rigidity, a positive Kernig sign, and flaccid paralysis of all four extremities. A CT scan confirmed the diagnosis of subarachnoid hemorrhage. Cerebral angiography revealed an aneurysm of the anterior communicating artery that had ruptured.

Treatable Diseases to Be Ruled Out
Bacterial meningitis
Temporal arteritis
Hypertensive encephalopathy

Comment: The illustration shows the blood in the subarachnoid space and the small aneurysm at the bifurcation of the internal carotid and anterior communicating arteries.

Synopsis: A subarachnoid hemorrhage is the most common presentation of a cerebral aneurysm. At least one-third of patients with subarachnoid hemorrhage die, and most of the other two-thirds become affected with some sort of disability. Diagnosis is made by CT and angiography. Definitive treatment is surgical clipping of the aneurysm at its neck, and this procedure is done within 48 to 72 hours of diagnosis. Intensive management of the subarachnoid hemorrhage includes methods to lower the intracranial pressure and supportive care as outlined in Appendix C.

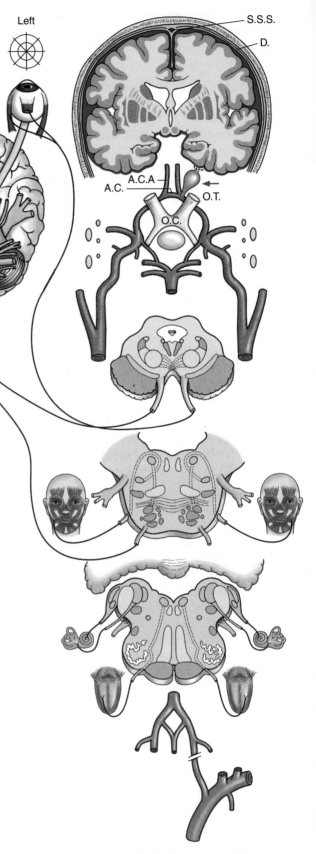

Figure 2. Brain: Subarachnoid Hemorrhage

SUBCLAVIAN STEAL SYNDROME

A 55-year-old white woman complained of frequent episodes of dizziness, ringing in the ears, and weakness and incoordination of her legs during the past 6 months. Some of these episodes were precipitated by exercise, particularly when she performed extensive workouts of her upper extremities.

Neurologic examination was unremarkable; however, it was noted that the patient had a diminished radial pulse and blood pressure in her left upper extremity. Four-vessel cerebral angiography demonstrated an occlusion of the left subclavian artery proximal to the vertebral artery with reverse flow of blood down the vertebral artery into the distal subclavian artery.

Treatable Diseases to Be Ruled Out
Epilepsy
Migraine
Vertebral-basilar insufficiency
Meniere's disease
Cardiac arrhythmia
Recurrent cerebral emboli
Space-occupying lesion
Hypoglycemia

Comment: The illustration demonstrates the occlusion of the left subclavian artery proximal to the exit of the vertebral artery and the reverse blood flow (*arrow*). The area of the medulla responsible for the symptoms is outlined.

Synopsis: This case is typical of vertebral-basilar insufficiency due to thrombosis or stenosis of the subclavian artery proximal to the vertebral artery. Vertebral-basilar insufficiency may also result from compression of the vertebral artery by osteophytes in the cervical spine and by atherosclerosis. Other symptoms of subclavian steal syndrome are visual disturbances, gaze paralysis, facial numbness or weakness, dysphagia, dysarthria, paresthesias, drop attacks, and loss of consciousness. The diagnosis is established by four-vessel cerebral angiography, but magnetic resonance angiography is also useful, especially in high-risk patients. Treatment is surgical endarterectomy if the obstruction is extracranial; otherwise, anticoagulants or antiplatelet drugs may be useful (see Appendix C). Many patients with this condition develop a completed stroke if they are left untreated.

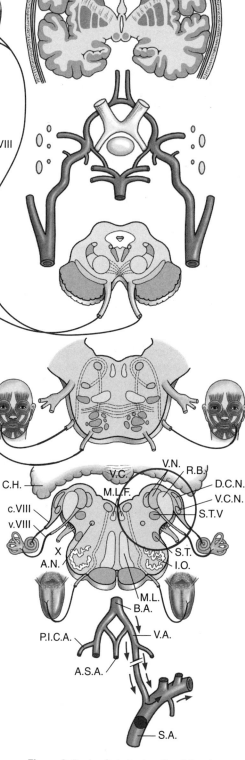

Figure 3. Brain: Subclavian Steal Syndrome

SUBDURAL HEMATOMA

A 28-year-old black man complained of constant bifrontal headache and blurred vision of 3 weeks' duration. He had mild intermittent frontal headaches for the past 8 months, and he said he had become irritable and "difficult to live with." For the past month, he was often extremely drowsy and sometimes slept 30 hours at a time. About 10 months previously, he fell from a moving vehicle and lacerated his scalp.

Neurologic examination revealed bilateral early papilledema, a dilated left pupil, and right hemiparesis. A CT scan demonstrated a left frontoparietal subdural hematoma, which was surgically evacuated.

Treatable Diseases to Be Ruled Out
General paresis
Toxic encephalopathy
Subdural empyema
Other space-occupying lesions of the cerebrum

Comment: The illustration shows the left frontoparietal hematoma compressing the brain and accounting for the right hemiparesis and early papilledema. The dilated pupil on the left is probably a result of mild compression of the oculomotor nerve by herniation of the uncus.

Synopsis: Subdural hematomas usually result from head trauma that causes the movement of the brain within the skull and tearing of the cerebral veins. Alcoholics and epileptics are particularly prone to such trauma, and the trauma may be trivial. These hematomas also may occur in the middle and posterior fossa or between the tentorium and occipital lobe. This case presents the typical symptoms and signs of a chronic subdural hematoma; patients with an acute subdural hematoma frequently lose consciousness or develop symptoms shortly after injury. Diagnosis is established by a CT scan. Treatment is surgical evacuation of the clot, unless the lesion is small, in which case the patient may be treated conservatively.

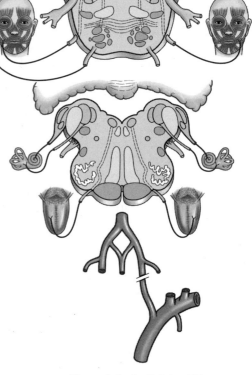

Figure 4. Brain: Subdural Hematoma

SPHENOID RIDGE MENINGIOMA

A 39-year-old black woman had a right frontal headache for the past 3 years. Eight months before she was admitted to the hospital, her husband noted that her right eye seemed to protrude. Three months later, she developed double vision.

Neurologic examination revealed right exophthalmos; papilledema; partial paralysis of right upward, downward, and medial gaze; a dilated right pupil that failed to respond to light or accommodation; and a diminished right corneal reflex. A CT scan confirmed the diagnosis. Thyroid function studies were normal.

Treatable Diseases to Be Ruled Out
Orbital cellulitis
Cavernous sinus thrombosis
Aneurysm of the circle of Willis
Graves' disease
Myasthenia gravis

Comment: The illustration shows the tumor on the longitudinal view compressing the third cranial nerve, causing paralysis of the right medial, upward, and downward gaze, and the trigeminal nerve, causing loss of the right corneal reflex.

Synopsis: The sphenoid ridge is another frequent location for meningiomas. These tumors produce a classical clinical syndrome that may easily be confused with Graves' disease, orbital cellulitis, or cavernous sinus thrombosis. Diagnosis is easily made by CT or MRI. Treatment and prognosis are discussed on page 148.

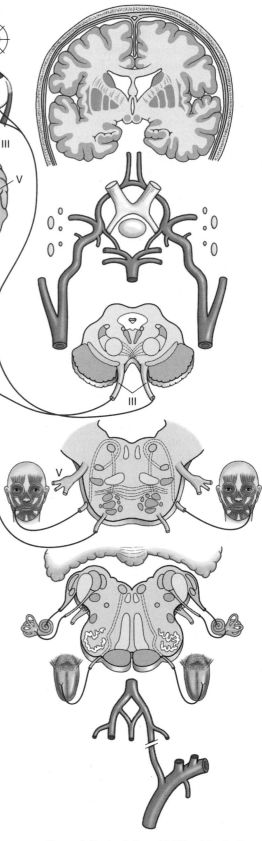

Figure 5. Brain: Sphenoid Ridge Meningioma

SYRINGOBULBIA

A 38-year-old woman had paroxysmal left facial pain for 2 years. Injections of lidocaine to the trigeminal nerve failed to relieve the pain. Two months before she was admitted to the hospital, she developed hoarseness and noisy breathing.

Neurologic examination disclosed absence of the left corneal reflex, hypalgesia of the left face and forehead, nystagmus on the left lateral gaze, deviation of the uvula to the right, atrophy and fasciculations of the left side of the tongue, loss of pain and temperature sensation over the right shoulder and arm, and an intention tremor of the left hand. An MRI confirmed the diagnosis. Spinal fluid examination and other laboratory and radiographic studies were normal.

Treatable Diseases to Be Ruled Out
Acoustic neuroma
Vertebral artery aneurysm
Platybasia
Neurosyphilis

Comment: The illustration shows the syrinx involving the descending tracts of the trigeminal nerve, causing the hypalgesia of the face; the hypoglossal nerve root, causing the atrophy and fasciculations of the tongue; the restiform body, causing the intention tremor of the left hand; and the spinothalamic tract, causing the loss of pain and temperature sensation in the right shoulder and arm.

Synopsis: See page 117.

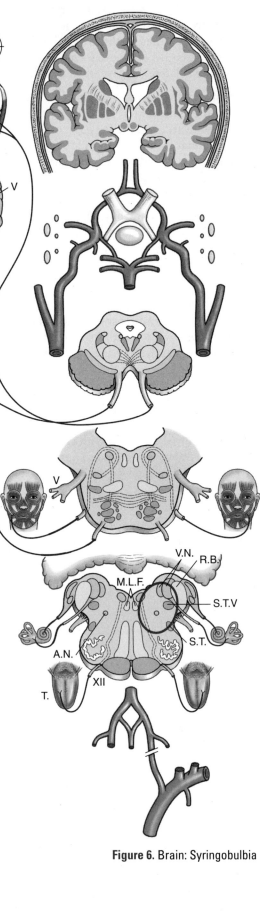

Figure 6. Brain: Syringobulbia

TRANSIENT ISCHEMIC ATTACK

A 55-year-old white man complained of intermittent loss of vision in his left eye associated with weakness of his right arm and hand.

Neurologic examination revealed a bruit over the left carotid artery. Carotid ultrasonography revealed an 85% occlusion of the left carotid artery at its bifurcation. Four-vessel cerebral angiography confirmed the diagnosis. The attacks subsided after the patient underwent carotid artery endarterectomy.

Treatable Diseases to Be Ruled Out
Cerebral embolism
Migraine
Optic neuritis
Space-occupying lesion of the brain
Epilepsy
Glaucoma

Comment: The illustration shows the partial occlusion of the left carotid artery (*arrow*) and associated monocular blindness and the involvement of the left cerebral hemisphere.

Synopsis: Transient ischemic attacks may occur in the carotid circulation, as in this case, or in the vertebral-basilar circulation. Transient monocular blindness and contralateral hemiparesis are common symptoms of carotid artery insufficiency, but hemianopsia, hemianesthesia, and aphasia may occur as well. Diagnosis is established by duplex ultrasonography and angiography, as in this case. Recurrent cerebral emboli may mimic the clinical picture, so a search for possible embolic sources is wise. Treatment for carotid insufficiency is surgical; however, if surgery is contraindicated, anticoagulation with warfarin sodium or antiplatelet agents may be beneficial (see Appendix C for dosages and treatment schedules). Balloon angioplasty may become an established alternative to bypass surgery and endarterectomy in the future.

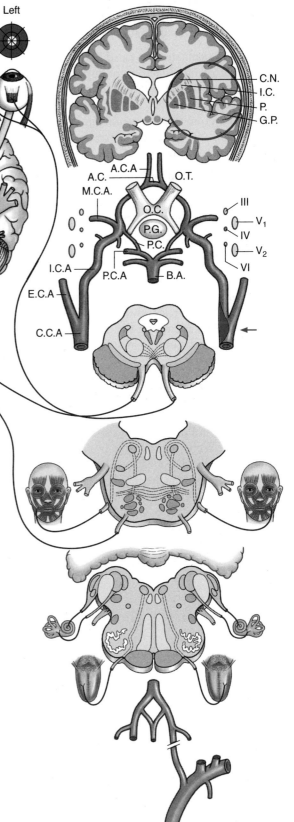

Figure 1. Brain: Transient Ischemic Attack

WEBER'S SYNDROME

A 54-year-old white woman had a sudden on-set of diplopia and weakness in her left arm and leg 2 days after she had a hysterectomy.

Neurologic examination revealed partial ptosis of the right eyelid; dilated right pupil; paresis of right upward, downward, and medial gaze; and left hemiparesis. An ECG showed atrial fibrillation. Four-vessel cerebral angiography was normal. A CT scan demonstrated the midbrain infarction.

Treatable Diseases to Be Ruled Out
Neurosyphilis
Migraine
Cerebral aneurysm
Vertebral-basilar insufficiency
Space-occupying lesion

Comment: The illustration shows the infarction involving the right pyramidal tract, causing the left hemiparesis, and the right oculomotor nerve root, causing the dilated pupil, ptosis, and paresis of upward, downward, and medial gaze.

Synopsis: This is a case of cerebral embolism in the basilar circulation due to chronic atrial fibrillation. See page 153 for a further discussion of the diagnosis and treatment of cerebral embolism. Cerebral emboli most commonly involve the carotid circulation. Weber's syndrome is just one of the many ways strokes in the basilar artery circulation may present. Infarction in the pons may present with abducens and facial palsy (Millard-Gubler syndrome). Obstruction of the top of the basilar artery may block the posterior cerebral arteries, causing cortical blindness and tunnel vision. Obstruction of the posterior inferior cerebellar artery is discussed on page 154. Obstruction of the branches of the vertebral basilar artery may present in many other ways.

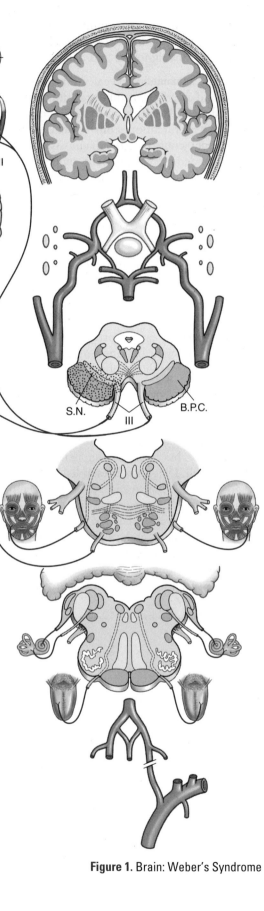

Figure 1. Brain: Weber's Syndrome

WERNICKE'S ENCEPHALOPATHY

A 44-year-old white man with alcoholism was admitted to the hospital in a semiconscious state.

Neurologic examination revealed dilated, fixed pupils and very little movement of the eyes in following light, although the patient was conscious enough to follow simple commands. The following morning, the patient was more alert, but examination revealed almost complete external ophthalmoplegia. Aside from an elevated blood alcohol level, laboratory and radiographic studies were normal. Within 30 hours of intravenous thiamine and multivitamins, the ophthalmoplegia had largely subsided.

Treatable Diseases to Be Ruled Out
Diabetic neuropathy
Myasthenia gravis
Cerebral aneurysm
Cavernous sinus thrombosis
Neurosyphilis
Tuberculous meningitis

Comment: The illustration reveals the involvement of the mammillary bodies and the periaqueductal gray matter of the hypothalamus, midbrain, and medulla, leading to oculomotor and abducens palsy and ophthalmoplegia.

Synopsis: Wernicke's encephalopathy is the result of thiamine deficiency and typically occurs in undernourished alcoholics, as does Korsakoff syndrome. The diagnosis is made by the response to intravenous thiamine, although MRI is supportive because it demonstrates the involvement of the periaqueductal gray matter and mammillary bodies. Treatment is thiamine (200 mg) given intravenously every 8 hours until the patient can take thiamine orally at 100 mg twice a day. A nutritious diet and multivitamin supplements are also essential. The prognosis for recovery is fair if the patient abstains from alcohol, but ataxia, amnesia, and nystagmus may persist.

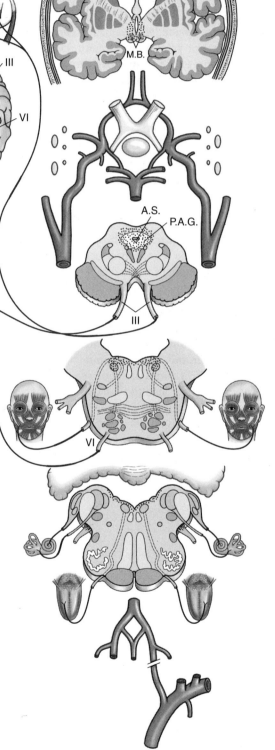

Figure 2. Brain: Wernicke's Encephalopathy

WILSON'S DISEASE

A 16-year-old white boy developed an increasing tremor and beating movements in his upper extremities during the 3 months before he was admitted to the hospital. His family also noted that he had unusual outbursts of laughter and difficulty swallowing food.

Neurologic examination revealed clownish facies; dysarthric speech; and tremor, rigidity, and rhythmic choreiform movements of the upper extremities. A Kayser-Fleischer ring was found in the limbus of the cornea on slit lamp examination. The diagnosis was confirmed by a low serum copper and ceruloplasmin level and high hepatic copper content on liver biopsy.

Treatable Diseases to Be Ruled Out
Phenothiazine toxicity
Hyperthyroidism

Comment: The illustration shows the diffuse involvement of the cortex, producing the dementia, and the involvement of the basal ganglia, causing the tremor, rigidity, and choreiform movements.

Synopsis: Wilson's disease is an autosomal recessive disorder involving a copper metabolism defect that causes neurologic and hepatic dysfunction. Diagnosis is established by low serum copper and ceruloplasmin levels and a high copper content in the hepatic tissue on liver biopsy. Hepatic involvement may lead to cirrhosis, splenomegaly, hematemesis, and liver failure. Treatment with penicillamine or tetrathiomolybdate may reverse the course of the disease (see Appendix C). Prognosis for complete or nearly complete recovery is good for patients treated early.

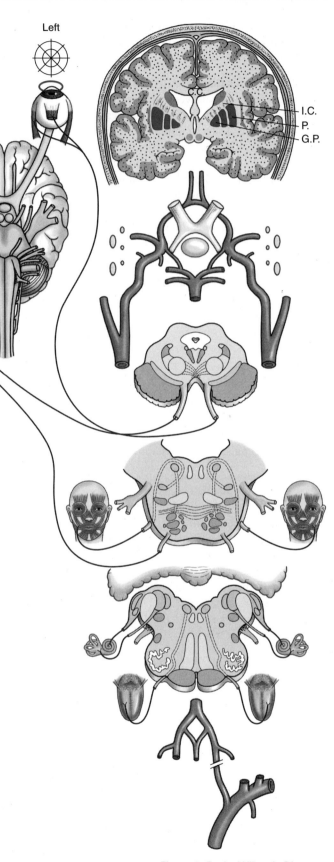

Figure 3. Brain: Wilson's Disease

APPENDIX A

ADDITIONAL SPECIAL EXAMINATIONS FOR EACH NEUROLOGIC SYMPTOM

1. Amnesia—Assessment of ability to interpret proverbial phrases and to follow simple and complex commands; evaluation of orientation to time, space, and politics; assessment of stereognosis; serial sevens; Draw-a-Person test; Minnesota Multiphasic Personality Inventory; Rorschach test; Mini-Mental Status Examination.
2. Anosmia—Smell testing with vanilla, mint, camphor, or ground coffee. (Test each nostril separately; if malingering is suspected, test with ammonia.)
3. Anxiety—Vital signs; Minnesota Multiphasic Personality Inventory.
4. Back pain—Straight leg–raising test; Patrick's test; femoral stretch test; rectal and vaginal examination; range of motion tests; measurement of leg, thigh, and calf length; assessment of heel and toe walking; assessment of power of extension of big toes.
5. Blindness—Testing of visual fields with tangent screen; evaluation of visual acuity, pupillary reactions, and hemianopic pupillary response; tonometry; slit lamp examination; ophthalmoscopic examination after administration of mydriatic drug.
6. Blurred vision—See Blindness.
7. Coma—Vital signs; auscultation of the heart; evaluation for breath odors, nuchal rigidity, Kernig's sign, limb resistance, limb withdrawal to pinprick, snout response to painful stimuli, and response to supraorbital ridge pressure; thorough general physical examination.
8. Convulsions—Examination of the tongue for lacerations; evaluation for signs of incontinence; examination of the skin for port-wine stains, café au lait spots, and other signs; evaluation of lesions and breath odors; auscultation of the heart; testing for nuchal rigidity; precipitation of petit mal via hyperventilation.
9. Deafness—Weber's test; Rinne test; otoscopic examination; audiogram; caloric tests; tympanogram; examination for vertical and horizontal nystagmus and Bruns' sign (see Appendix D, Glossary).
10. Delirium—See Coma.
11. Delusions—See Amnesia.
12. Depression—See Amnesia.
13. Difficulty urinating—Rectal examination, including assessment of sphincter control; vaginal examination; assessment of superficial abdominal and cremasteric reflexes; catheterization for residual urine.
14. Diplopia—Red-glass test; measurement of eyeballs for exophthalmos; examination for nystagmus; Tensilon test.
15. Dizziness—Otoscopic examination; wristwatch test; Weber's test; Rinne test; audiogram; caloric test; examination for nystagmus; evaluation for past-pointing sign and Romberg's sign; Hallpike maneuvers (see Appendix D, Glossary); hyperventilation to duplicate symptoms; evaluation of carotid and radial pulses; auscultation for bruits; auscultation of the heart; thorough general physical examination.
16. Dystonia—Assessment for Kayser-Fleischer ring; Mini-Mental Status Examination.
17. Extremity pain, lower—Straight leg–raising test; Patrick's test; testing for Homans' sign; evaluation of femoral, popliteal, and tibial pulses; hip and knee joint range-of-motion tests; examination for torn meniscus, etc.; testing for hot and cold sensation.
18. Extremity pain, upper—Cervical compression test; Spurling's test; shoulder, elbow, and wrist joint range-of-motion tests; testing for Tinel's sign at the elbow and wrist; Adson's test for scalenus anticus syndrome; stellate ganglion block; auscultation for bruit over the subclavian artery; evaluation of hot and cold sensation.
19. Eye pain—Funduscopic examination; tonometry; slip lamp examination; visual field examination; assessment of visual acuity; red-glass test.
20. Face pain—Evaluation by tapping the teeth and exits of branches of trigeminal nerves; transillumination of the sinuses; nasopharyngeal examination; examination of the temporomandibular joint for crepitus; evaluation of the bite for malocclusion, jaw strength, and jaw jerk; corneal reflex test; assessment of hot and cold sensation.
21. Hallucinations—See Amnesia.
22. Headache—Compression of the superficial temporal artery to determine whether headache is relieved; compression of the bilateral jugular vein to determine whether headache is relieved; examination of the superficial temporal artery for tenderness or enlargement; examination for nuchal rigidity; auscultation for bruits over the neck, head, and orbit; transillumination of the sinuses; tonometry; sumatriptan trial; nitroglycerin provocation gr. 1/150.
23. Hip pain—Patrick's test; femoral stretch test; straight leg–raising test; lidocaine injection to the greater trochanter bursa to assess pain relief.
24. Hoarseness—Ear, nose, and throat examination; indirect or direct laryngoscopic examination; auscultation of the heart and lungs; gag reflex test; examination of the palate and uvula for position and movement; Tensilon test.
25. Hypersomnia—See Amnesia.

26. Impotence—Rectal examination, including rectal sphincter control; examination of superficial abdominal and cremasteric reflexes; penile blood pressure test; examination of femoral pulses and other peripheral pulses; examination for secondary sex characteristics; examination for the presence of residual urine.

27. Incontinence—Rectal and vaginal examination; evaluation of superficial abdominal and cremasteric reflexes; evaluation of rectal sphincter tone and control; examination for the presence of residual urine.

28. Insomnia—Mental Status Examination; Minnesota Multiphasic Personality Inventory.

29. Memory loss—Assessment of orientation to time, space, and politics; evaluation of attention span; assessment of ability to interpret proverbial phrases and to follow simple and complex commands; serial sevens; reading, writing, and arithmetic tests; assessment of stereognosis; evaluation of sucking and grasp reflexes; examination of visual fields; evaluation of sense of smell; Mini-Mental Status Examination.

30. Neck pain—Cervical compression test; Spurling's test; range of motion test; examination for nuchal rigidity; examination for Kernig's sign; palpation of thyroid and nerve roots.

31. Nightmares—Mental Status Examination; Minnesota Multiphasic Personality Inventory; Rorschach test.

32. Paresthesias—See Extremity pain, lower, and Extremity pain, upper.

33. Photophobia—See Headache.

34. Restless legs syndrome—Examination for tremor, rigidity, athetosis, and chorea; examination of the thyroid for enlargement; evaluation of peripheral pulses.

35. Scotoma—See Blindness.

36. Sleep apnea—See Amnesia.

37. Sleepwalking—See Amnesia.

38. Syncope—Auscultation of the chest for carotid bruit, heart murmurs, and arrhythmias; evaluation of blood pressure with patient lying down then immediately standing; evaluation of all peripheral pulses; evaluation of blood pressure in each extremity; examination for tongue lacerations; determination of response to hyperventilation.

39. Tinnitus—See Deafness.

40. Weakness of one or more extremities—Testing for Gordon, Oppenheim, and Chaddock signs; examination of superficial abdominal and cremasteric reflexes; evaluation of rectal tone and control; measurement of muscle mass; Tensilon test; testing for Rossolimo's sign; testing for Hoffmann and Tromner reflexes; examination for clonus and fasciculations; testing for myotonic reflex; assessment of muscle fatigability.

APPENDIX B

LABORATORY WORKUP OF NEUROLOGIC DISEASES

Acoustic neuroma—Electronystagmography, MRI with gadolinium enhancement, angiography, combined myelography and CT.

Acquired immunodeficiency disease—Human immunodeficiency virus antibody titer.

Alcoholism—Blood alcohol level, liver function tests, liver biopsy.

Alzheimer's disease—CT or MRI, cisternography, psychometric testing.

Amyotrophic lateral sclerosis—Electromyography, clinical diagnosis.

Barbiturate intoxication—Urine drug screen, EEG.

Basilar artery thrombosis or insufficiency—MRI, magnetic resonance angiography, four-vessel cerebral angiography.

Bell's palsy—CT of mastoid process and petrous portion of the temporal bone to rule out serious pathology, electromyography.

Brachial plexus neuropathy—Nerve conduction velocity studies, electromyography, somatosensory evoked potentials.

Brain tumor—MRI preferred over CT.

Carotid artery stenosis or insufficiency—Carotid duplex scan, magnetic resonance angiography, four-vessel cerebral angiography.

Carpal tunnel syndrome—Nerve conduction velocity studies, electromyography.

Cavernous sinus thrombosis—CT, magnetic resonance angiography, blood cultures.

Cerebellar abscess—CT or MRI, blood cultures.

Cerebral aneurysm—MRI, magnetic resonance angiography, four-vessel cerebral angiography.

Cerebral embolism—MRI, ECG, echocardiography, blood cultures, carotid duplex scan.

Cerebral hemorrhage—CT, MRI, hypertensive workup later.

Cerebral thrombosis—CT, MRI, consider arteriography later.

Cervical spondylosis—Radiography of cervical spine, MRI, myelography, electromyography.

Compression fracture—CT, MRI.

Encephalitis—Viral isolation from spinal fluid, serologic test.

Epidural abscess—CT or MRI.

Epidural hematoma—Radiography of the skull, CT or MRI.

Epilepsy—EEG (awake and asleep), MRI, ambulatory EEG monitoring.

Familial tremor—Clinical diagnosis.

Friedreich's ataxia—Clinical diagnosis.

General paresis—Venereal Disease Research Laboratory (VDRL) test, blood fluorescent treponemal antibody absorption test (FTA-ABS), spinal fluid FTA-ABS.

Glioblastoma—CT or MRI.

Guillain-Barré syndrome—Spinal tap, nerve conduction velocity studies, electromyography.

Herniated disc—CT or MRI (MRI is the procedure of choice in cervical disc disease), nerve conduction velocity studies, electromyography.

Herpes zoster—Serologic tests (but clinical diagnosis is usually sufficient).

Histamine cephalgia—Histamine test, response to sumatriptan.

Huntington's chorea—MRI, clinical diagnosis.

Lead intoxication—Blood and urine lead level, urine delta-aminolevulinic acid and coproporphyrin levels, blood free erythrocyte protoporphyrin level, radiography of long bones.

Medulloblastoma—CT or MRI.

Meniere's disease—Audiogram, caloric test, electronystagmography.

Meningioma—CT or MRI.

Meningitis—Blood cultures; spinal fluid examination, culture, and India ink staining.

Migraine—CT to rule out serious pathology, response to sumatriptan.

Multiple sclerosis—MRI of the brain and spinal cord; spinal tap; somatosensory, visual, and brainstem auditory evoked potentials.

Muscular dystrophy—Electromyography, muscle biopsy.

Myasthenia gravis—Acetylcholine receptor antibody titer, Tensilon test, electromyography, search for thymoma.

Narcolepsy—Polysomnography.

Neurosyphilis—Venereal Disease Research Laboratory (VDRL) test, blood and spinal fluid fluorescent treponemal antibody absorption tests.

Optic neuritis—Visual fields, MRI, spinal tap.

Parkinson's disease—Clinical diagnosis.

Peripheral neuropathy—Nerve conduction velocity studies, electromyography, spinal tap, heavy metal screen, glucose tolerance test, human immunodeficiency virus antibody titer, antinuclear antibody test, urine porphobilinogen level, muscle biopsy.

Pernicious anemia—Serum vitamin B_{12} level, Schilling test, complete blood count, bone marrow examination.

Peroneal muscular atrophy—Nerve conduction velocity studies, electromyography, nerve biopsy.

Pituitary tumor—CT or MRI, endocrine diagnosis.

Progressive muscular atrophy—Electromyography, clinical diagnosis.

Sleep apnea—Polysomnography.

Spinal cord tumor—MRI of the spine, bone scan for metastasis.

Subarachnoid hemorrhage—CT, spinal tap, angiography.

Subdural hematoma—CT or MRI.

Syringomyelia—CT or MRI.

Temporal arteritis—Erythrocyte sedimentation rate, artery biopsy.

Thoracic outlet syndrome—Nerve conduction velocity studies, angiography, radiography of the cervical spine.

Transient ischemic attack—Carotid duplex scan, echocardiography, ECG, four-vessel cerebral angiography.

Trigeminal neuralgia—Clinical diagnosis.

Werdnig-Hoffmann disease—Electromyography, clinical diagnosis.

Wernicke's encephalopathy—Therapeutic trial of intravenous thiamine.

Wilson's disease—Slit lamp examination, serum copper and ceruloplasmin levels, liver biopsy.

APPENDIX C

TREATMENT OF NEUROLOGIC DISEASES

Acoustic neuroma—Surgery is indicated.

Alzheimer's disease—No specific treatment is available. Supportive care includes a high-vitamin diet, sedation, and antidepressants. Donepezil (5 to 10 mg daily [Aricept; Pfizer, New York, NY]) has improved cognitive function over a 30-week period. Tacrine (120 to 160 mg daily [Cognex; West-ward Pharmaceutical Corp., Eatontown, NJ]) may also improve cognition. When using tacrine, monitor liver functions carefully.

Amyotrophic lateral sclerosis—Treatment is supportive as no specific therapy is available.

Basilar artery thrombosis or insufficiency
1. Confirm the diagnosis with CT to rule out hemorrhage and with magnetic resonance angiography or four-vessel cerebral angiography.
2. If the patient is seen within 3 hours of onset of symptoms, consider intra-arterial thrombolysis or intravenous tissue plasminogen activator. Consult a neurologist for guidance.
3. If the patient is seen 3 hours or more after onset and a definite thrombosis is noted and there is no hypertension or intracranial bleeding, begin anticoagulation with heparin, 5000 to 10,000 units loading dose, followed by 1000 to 1500 units hourly based on partial thromboplastin levels. Follow up with sodium warfarin (2 to 10 mg daily) orally for 6 to 12 months or longer if there is a repeat of the attack.
4. If the patient has hypertension, control the hypertension and initiate antiplatelet therapy with aspirin (325 mg daily) and/or ticlopidine (250 mg twice daily with food). Monitor liver function.

Bell's palsy
1. Give prednisone (60 mg daily) for 1 to 3 weeks, then gradually taper the dosage. In addition, administer acyclovir (200 mg five times daily) for 10 days.
2. Alternatively, give adrenocorticotropic hormone gel (80 units daily) for 3 days, then taper the dosage over 10-day period.
3. Have the patient keep his or her eyes moist with an eye patch and artificial tears.
4. Electrical stimulation of the facial muscles may be needed if recovery is prolonged. Consult a physiotherapist.

Brachial plexus neuropathy—Treatment is supportive, with a nutritious diet, high doses of vitamin B supplements, and physiotherapy.

Brain tumor—Surgery, radiation, or chemotherapy is indicated, depending on the tumor type. Consult a neurosurgeon and oncologist.

Carotid artery stenosis or insufficiency
1. Consult a cardiovascular surgeon for carotid endarterectomy or bypass surgery.

2. If surgery is not feasible, consider medical treatment as outlined under "Basilar artery thrombosis or insufficiency."

Carpal tunnel syndrome
1. Try vitamin B_6 (pyridoxine; 100 mg three times daily) for 6 to 12 weeks.
2. If pyridoxine is ineffective, try an injection of triamcinolone suspension (20 mg) and lidocaine (0.5 mL) into the carpal tunnel. Experience is required for the administration of this therapy.
3. If the result is poor, consider carpal tunnel release. Consult a neurosurgeon or orthopedic surgeon.

Cavernous sinus thrombosis
1. Initiate treatment with intravenous penicillin G (2 million units every 2 hours) and ceftriaxone (2 g every 12 hours).
2. If the patient is sensitive to penicillin, administer ceftriaxone, chloramphenicol, or vancomycin.
3. Base antibiotic choice on spinal fluid culture results.
4. The use of anticoagulants is controversial. Consult a neurologist for guidance.

Cerebellar and cerebral abscess
1. Look for the primary source of infection (e.g., sinuses, mastoid process).
2. A small abscess may be treated with intravenous aqueous penicillin G (20 to 24 million units daily) and metronidazole (750 mg three times daily). Alternatively, add chloramphenicol (1 to 1.5 g intravenously every 6 hours). Continue treatment for 4 to 6 weeks.
3. If the results are poor, consult a neurosurgeon for immediate drainage and continue antibiotic therapy.
4. For a large abscess, consult a neurosurgeon for immediate surgery while starting the patient on antibiotics.
5. When culture results return from the laboratory, antibiotics may be adjusted accordingly.

Cerebral aneurysm
1. If the aneurysm has not ruptured, surgery is indicated.
2. For a ruptured aneurysm, see "Subarachnoid hemorrhage."

Cerebral embolism
1. Look for embolism's source.
2. If the patient has a significant neurologic deficit, treat cerebral edema with an osmotic solution such as mannitol before starting anticoagulants.
3. If the deficit is mild to moderate, administer intravenous heparin, 5000 to 10,000 units loading dose, followed by 1000 to 1500 units per hour to maintain a partial thromboplastin time of 1.5 to 2.5 times the control.
4. After the acute stage, treat the patient with warfarin sodium for 6 to 9 months to prevent a recurrence.

Cerebral hemorrhage

1. Provide supportive care.
2. Control hypertension with nifedipine (10 to 20 mg orally [chewable]) or labetalol (2 mg per minute intravenously to a maximum of 200 mg), but do not treat too aggressively.
3. Control cerebral edema with mannitol (0.5 to 1.0 g/kg intravenously over 15 to 30 minutes, then 25 to 50 g every 4 to 6 hours) to keep osmolality above 300 osmoles of solute per kilogram of solvent.
4. Consult a neurosurgeon for the feasibility of surgical evacuation.

Cerebral thrombosis—See "Basilar artery thrombosis and insufficiency."

Cervical spondylosis

1. Treat conservatively with cervical traction (in horizontal position) beginning at 10 lb (4.54 kg) for 1 to 2 hours a day, gradually increasing to 15 lb (6.81 kg) over a 4- to 6-week period.
2. Other conservative measures may be tried, including cervical collar, physiotherapy, muscle relaxants, and nonsteroidal anti-inflammatory drugs.
3. If conservative measures fail or significant nerve root or cord compression is evident, consult a neurosurgeon for immediate decompression.

Compression fracture—Surgery is indicated.

Chronic demyelination neuropathy—Treat with prednisone (60 to 80 mg daily over 6 to 8 weeks, then gradually taper), plasmapheresis, and immunoglobulin.

Encephalitis

1. Provide supportive care.
2. Give anticonvulsants to control seizures.
3. Control increased intracranial pressure.
4. For herpes simplex virus encephalitis, give acyclovir (10 mg/kg every 8 hours) for 10 to 14 days. Look for nephrotoxicity. Encephalitis caused by influenza A can be treated with amantadine.

Epidural abscess—Surgical evacuation and antibiotics are indicated. See also "Cerebellar and cerebral abscess."

Epidural hematoma—Surgery is indicated.

Epilepsy; grand mal, focal, cortical, and complex partial seizures

1. Try monotherapy with phenytoin (100 to 600 mg daily), carbamazepine (200 to 1200 mg/day in divided doses), or valproate (250 to 1250 mg/day in divided doses). Monitor blood levels.
2. If seizures are in poor control, push the drug to maximum blood levels.
3. If control is still poor, try combinations of phenytoin, carbamazepine, and valproate.
4. If poor control continues, try a second-line drug such as clonazepam (0.5 to 1.5 mg three times daily), gabapentin (900 to 1200 mg daily in divided doses), or lamotrigine (300 to 500 mg daily).
5. If poor control continues, refer the patient to a special center for surgery of the cortical focus.

Epilepsy; petit mal seizures

1. If the patient has petit mal seizures only, first try ethosuximide (250 to 1250 mg daily in two divided doses).
2. If the patient has mixed seizures, try valproate (250 to 1250 mg daily in divided doses).
3. If the first or second treatment above elicits a poor response, give phenobarbital (30 to 120 mg daily in a single dose or divided doses) or clonazepam (0.5 to 5.0 mg daily in divided doses).
4. If the response is still poor, consult a neurologist.

Familial tremor

1. Propranolol (80 mg every 12 hours [Inderal LA; Wyeth Pharmaceuticals, Philadelphia, PA]).
2. If beta-blocker therapy is ineffective, try clonazepam (0.5 to 1.5 mg three times daily). Watch out for drowsiness.
3. Alternatively, try primidone (125 mg daily, increasing gradually to 250 mg three times daily [Mysoline; AstraZeneca, Waltham, MA]).

Friedreich's ataxia—Provide supportive care; no specific treatment is available.

General paresis—See "Neurosyphilis."

Glioblastoma—Treatment is with surgery, radiation, and/or chemotherapy in consultation with a neurosurgeon and oncologist.

Guillain-Barré syndrome

1. Hospitalization and supportive care are indicated. Look for respiratory paralysis, and treat if present.
2. Try plasmapheresis.
3. If plasmapheresis is unsuccessful, try high-dose immunoglobulin therapy (2 g/kg) over a 5-day period.
4. Corticosteroids are not of proven value but may be tried.

Herniated disc

1. If there is no definite weakness or atrophy of the extremities and no signs of spinal cord or cauda equina compression, conservative therapy in the form of muscle relaxants, anti-inflammatory drugs, and physiotherapy may be tried first.
2. If pain and disability persist after several weeks of conservative therapy, discectomy or laminectomy is indicated.
3. If there is definite weakness, atrophy, or spinal cord or cauda equina compression either in the beginning or during the course of conservative therapy, surgical intervention must be recommended.

Herpes zoster

1. Give acyclovir (800 mg five times daily) for 7 to 10 days or valacyclovir HCl (1000 mg) for 7 days.
2. Treat postherpetic neuralgia with a tricyclic antidepressant such as amitriptyline (25 to 75 mg three times daily) or nerve blocks. Transcutaneous electrical nerve stimulation may be effective.
3. Treat disseminated infection in immunocompromised patients with acyclovir (5 to 10 mg/kg intravenously every 8 hours). Consult an infectious disease specialist for guidance.

Histamine cephalgia

1. Treat acute attacks with sumatriptan (6 mg subcutaneously). Oxygen and parenteral narcotics may be given if sumatriptan fails.
2. To prevent attacks, give prednisone (1 mg/kg daily in divided doses for 7 to 10 days, then taper dosage). Therapy may need to continue for 4 to 6 weeks.
3. Methysergide (2 to 4 mg three times daily) may also be used to prevent attacks. Continue treatment for 2 weeks after attacks have subsided. Watch for retroperitoneal fibrosis.

Huntington's chorea

1. No specific cure is available.
2. Treat chorea with haloperidol (0.5 to 2.0 mg three times daily) or tetrabenazine (25 to 50 mg three times daily). Consult a neurologist for guidance.
3. Rigidity may be treated with baclofen (10 mg daily, gradually increasing to 80 mg daily).

Lead intoxication

1. Administer calcium disodium edetate (EDTA; up to 1.5 g per square meter of body surface, intravenously).

2. Alternatively, penicillamine (20 to 40 mg/kg daily) or dimercaprol (up to 12 to 24 mg/kg daily) may be given.
3. In cases of acute encephalopathy, a combination of EDTA and dimercaprol may be required.

Medulloblastoma—Surgery, radiation, or chemotherapy is indicated; consult a neurosurgeon and oncologist.

Meniere's disease
1. Treat acute attacks with meclizine (12.5 to 25 mg three times daily). Treat vomiting with prochlorperazine (12.5 mg intramuscularly). Alternatively, a transdermal scopolamine patch may be applied behind the ear.
2. To prevent attacks, a diuretic such as hydrochlorothiazide (50 mg daily) may be tried along with a potassium supplement. Triamterene in combination with hydrochlorothiazide also may be tried.
3. If the above treatment is ineffective, try a 14-day course of prednisone (40 to 60 mg daily for 1 week, then taper the dosage).
4. Encourage the patient to avoid cigarettes, caffeine, and alcohol.
5. If medical therapy is not successful, a shunting procedure or surgical destruction of the labyrinth may be necessary.

Meningioma—Surgery is indicated.

Meningitis, bacterial
1. Begin treatment with penicillin G (2 million units intravenously every 2 hours) along with ceftriaxone (2 g intravenously every 12 hours). If the patient is penicillin sensitive, give chloramphenicol (1 to 1.5 g intravenously every 6 hours) or vancomycin (500 mg intravenously every 6 hours; consult an infectious disease specialist for guidance).
2. Once the organism has been identified by cultures, choose the appropriate antibiotic for the organism involved.

Migraine
1. Treat acute attacks first with sumatriptan (25 to 100 mg orally or 3 to 6 mg subcutaneously). The oral dosage may be repeated once in 2 to 4 hours, but give no more than 200 mg in a 24-hour period. Alternatively, sumatriptan nasal spray may be used (5 mg in each nostril; repeat once in 2 to 4 hours).
2. If the response to sumatriptan is poor, try prochlorperazine (5 to 10 mg intravenously) and/or diphenhydramine (50 to 100 mg slowly intravenously).
3. If the response is still poor, consult a neurologist and consider admitting the patient to the hospital for intravenous fluids, corticosteroids, and oxygen.
4. To prevent migraines:
   a. A tyramine-free diet, with elimination of nuts, chocolate, and, particularly, aged cheeses, may be helpful.
   b. In children, try cyproheptadine (2 to 4 mg four times daily) or phenytoin (50 to 300 mg daily). Consult a neurologist.
   c. In women with menstrual migraine, try a combination of ergotamine and a nonsteroidal anti-inflammatory drug such as naproxen (500 mg twice daily). Alternatively, medroxyprogesterone (150 mg intramuscularly) may be given every 3 to 4 months to suppress menstruation. Consult a gynecologist.
   d. Migraines in most adults can be controlled with a long-acting beta-blocker, such as atenolol (25 to 100 mg daily) or metoprolol (50 to 200 mg daily), or with a tricyclic antidepressant, such as nortriptyline (10 to 50 mg at bedtime), either alone or combined with a beta-blocker. Other preparations that may be used include phenytoin (200 to 400 mg daily), valproate (250 to 1250 mg daily in divided doses), and methysergide (2 to 4 mg three times a day). Consult a neurologist for guidance.

Multiple sclerosis
1. Treat acute attacks with methylprednisolone (20 to 40 mg four times daily, or 1 g daily, intravenously for 5 to 7 days, then taper dosage).
2. Patients with the relapsing and remitting form of the disease may reduce the relapse rate by taking interferon beta-1a (once weekly intramuscularly or every other day subcutaneously).
3. Glatiramer acetate (daily subcutaneously) may also be effective.
4. The patient should be on a low-fat diet and should avoid milk products.
5. Daily doses of sublingual vitamin B_{12} or weekly intramuscular injections of B_{12} also seem to reduce exacerbations.
6. Spasticity may be reduced with baclofen (10 to 120 mg four times daily).

Muscular dystrophy—No definitive treatment is available, but prednisone (0.75 mg/kg daily orally) may sustain muscle strength for up to 3 years in Duchenne's muscular dystrophy. The myotonia of myotonic dystrophy may be reduced by phenytoin (up to 300 mg daily orally).

Myasthenia gravis
1. Look for thymoma, and consider thymectomy in all patients over the age of puberty.
2. First, administer treatment with an anticholinesterase drug, such as pyridostigmine (60 mg three to five times daily; may be increased to 80 mg four times daily). Evaluate the need for larger doses with the edrophonium (Tensilon) response test.
3. If the response to anticholinesterase drugs is poor, initiate corticosteroids. Prednisone may be started at a dosage of 15 to 25 mg daily then gradually increased until a response occurs. Continue the response dosage for 1 to 3 months, then gradually reduce to alternate-day therapy. Hospitalization may be required during the initial period of corticosteroid administration.
4. An immunosuppressant drug, such as azathioprine or cyclophosphamide, may be tried next. Consult an oncologist.
5. Treat myasthenic crises with immediate hospitalization, intubation, and artificial respiration under the care of an anesthesiologist and neurologist. Stop all anticholinesterase drugs, and perform the Tensilon test. Plasmapheresis and intravenous immunoglobulin should be considered.

Narcolepsy
1. Try pemoline (Cylert; Abbott Laboratories, Abbott Park, IL [37.5 to 75 mg daily]).
2. If pemoline is ineffective, try methylphenidate (Ritalin; Novartis, East Hanover, NJ [10 to 20 mg daily]).
3. If pemoline and methylphenidate are ineffective, try amphetamines.
4. Treat cataplexy with imipramine (25 mg three times daily) or other tricyclic antidepressant.

Neurosyphilis
1. Administer aqueous penicillin G (12 to 14 million units daily intravenously for 14 days).
2. Alternatively, patients may be given benzathine penicillin (2.4 million units weekly intramuscularly for 3 weeks).
3. Patients who are sensitive to penicillin may be either desensitized and treated or given tetracycline HCl (500 mg four times daily orally for 30 days).

Normal pressure hydrocephalus—Surgery is indicated.

Optic neuritis
1. Administer intravenous methylprednisolone (1000 mg daily for 3 days), then switch to oral methylprednisolone (1 mg/kg daily in divided doses for 10 days, then taper dosage over a 3-week period).
2. Alternatively, adrenocorticotropic hormone gel may be given intramuscularly in doses of 80 units daily for 4 days, then 40 units daily for 4 days, then 20 units daily for 4 days.

Parkinson's disease
1. Begin treatment with a combination of carbidopa and levodopa (Sinemet; Merck & Co., West Point, PA [25/100 mg three times daily]), gradually increasing the dosage until a good response is achieved. Once optimum control is achieved, the patient may be switched to a controlled-release preparation.
2. If the response to Sinemet deteriorates, try pergolide, ropinirole, or pramipexole. Pergolide may be given in dosages of 0.75 to 5.0 mg daily. Ropinirole is begun with a dose of 0.25 mg three times a day, increased gradually until clinical success is achieved or until a total dose of 24 mg is reached (consult a neurologist for guidance). Pramipexole is given initially at a dose of 0.125 mg three times a day and is gradually increased until clinical success is achieved or a dose of 1.5 mg three times a day is reached (consult a neurologist for guidance).
3. Selegiline may be tried, although it has failed to provide a long-term neuroprotective effect.
4. If the response to the drugs mentioned above becomes ineffective or the patient is young, consider referral to a neurosurgeon for adrenal medullary transplantation or stereotactic surgery.

Peripheral neuropathy
1. Confirm the cause and treat it.
2. For treatment of Guillain-Barré syndrome, see page 170.
3. For treatment of lead neuropathy, see page 170.
4. For porphyria, administer an intravenous glucose infusion of hemin. Consult a neurologist.
5. For diabetic neuropathy, control blood sugar, improve nutrition, and provide a high-dosage vitamin B supplement. Treat painful neuropathy with tricyclic antidepressants, anticonvulsants, or topical capsaicin.
6. For inherited neuropathy, no treatment is available.
7. For nutritional neuropathy, give a combination of thiamine and niacin (50 mg each three times daily) and pyridoxine (100 mg three times daily) and encourage the patient to eat a healthy diet and to take a multivitamin supplement.
8. For treatment of chronic demyelinating inflammatory neuropathy, see page 170.

Pernicious anemia
1. Initiate treatment with vitamin B_{12} (1000 µg intramuscularly twice weekly for 2 months, then twice monthly for life).
2. Do not give folic acid until after the first month of vitamin B_{12} therapy.

Peroneal muscular atrophy—Treatment is supportive as no specific therapy is available.

Pituitary tumor—Surgery is indicated.

Sleep apnea—Consult a pulmonologist.

Spinal cord tumor—Surgery is indicated.

Subarachnoid hemorrhage
1. Treat the source of the hemorrhage (aneurysm) with early surgery, as long as the patient is stable. Early surgery is no longer believed to produce or aggravate cerebral ischemia and infarction.
2. Control hypertension, cerebral edema, and increased intracranial pressure as outlined under "Cerebral hemorrhage" on page 170.
3. If there is a progressive neurologic deficit due to ischemia, administer the calcium channel blocker nimodipine (60 mg every 4 hours for 21 days).
4. Hypervolemic therapy may be tried with an infusion of plasma protein and monitoring of pulmonary capillary wedge pressure. Consult a neurologist.
5. Papaverine infusion may also control vasospasm.

Subdural hematoma—Surgery is indicated.

Syringomyelia—For mild cases with very slow deterioration, no treatment is required. If the disease is progressing rapidly, a shunting procedure or reconstruction of the subarachnoid space may be indicated. Consult a neurosurgeon.

Temporal arteritis
1. Treat acute attacks with prednisone (30 mg twice daily for 1 to 2 weeks, then taper dosage over a 4- to 6-week period).
2. Continue a maintenance dose of prednisone (7.5 to 10 mg daily) for 1 to 2 years to prevent relapse.

Thoracic outlet syndrome
1. Conservative treatment with shoulder shrug exercises and physiotherapy is indicated. Adjustment of posture may help.
2. Consult an orthopedic surgeon for surgical evaluation.

Transient ischemic attack—Administer anticoagulation or antiplatelet therapy as outlined under "Basilar artery thrombosis or insufficiency" on page 169. Consider surgical evaluation for large-vessel disease.

Trigeminal neuralgia
1. Administer carbamazepine (100 mg twice daily), increasing the dosage until a response is achieved or a maximum dosage of 400 mg twice daily is reached.
2. Alternatively, phenytoin (300 to 600 mg daily) may be tried.
3. If carbamazepine and phenytoin do not produce a successful response, try baclofen (10 to 20 mg twice daily).
4. If drug treatment is not successful, consult a neurosurgeon.

Werdnig-Hoffmann disease—No treatment is available.

Wernicke's encephalopathy—Administer intravenous thiamine (200 mg every 8 hours) until the patient can take thiamine orally (100 mg twice daily).

Wilson's disease
1. Institute dietary measures to reduce copper intake.
2. Initial treatment to lower copper levels to normal is tetrathiomolybdate (60 to 300 mg daily divided into six doses).
3. Alternatively, trientine (250 mg four times daily) may be given.
4. Also, penicillamine (600 to 3000 mg daily) has been given, but toxic side effects have been noted in up to 25% of patients.
5. Once serum copper is brought to a normal level, zinc acetate (50 mg three times daily) may be given for maintenance.

APPENDIX D

GLOSSARY AND BIBLIOGRAPHY

Glossary

Adie's syndrome. Tonic pupil together with the absence of the patellar reflex.

Altitudinopsia. A defect of the upper or lower half of the visual field.

Ankle clonus. A series of rhythmic, hyperactive ankle jerks produced by forcible and brisk dorsiflexion of the foot.

Apraxia. Inability to perform purposeful motions.

Astasia-abasia. Apparent inability to walk or stand caused by some mental conflict.

Astereognosis. Inability to recognize objects by the sense of touch.

Ataxia. Incoordination of muscular action.

Athetosis. Recurrent, slow, and continual change in the position of the fingers and toes or any part of the body.

Babinski's sign. Extension of the great toe with fanning of the other toes on stimulation of the sole of the foot.

Babinski-Weil test. A test to determine vestibular and cerebellar function, performed by having the patient walk forward or backward 10 or more times with the eyes closed. In cerebellar or vestibular disease, the patient deviates to the side of the lesion.

Benedikt's syndrome. Contralateral hemianesthesia and involuntary choreiform movements and homolateral oculomotor paresis in occlusion of the paramedian basilar branch that supplies the red nucleus and the medial lemniscus.

Brudzinski's sign. A sign of meningeal irritation in which raising the recumbent patient's head causes involuntary flexion of the thighs.

Bruns' syndrome. A form of episodic vertigo, headache, disturbance of vision, and feeling of blacking out on flexion or extension of the head seen in posterior fossa tumors.

Café au lait spots. Areas on the skin of a "coffee with cream" color, often associated with von Recklinghausen's disease.

Caloric test. A test for vestibular function performed by placing water at various temperatures in the external auditory meatus and observing for nystagmus.

Chaddock's sign. Extension of the great toe and fanning of the other toes on stroking the lateral malleolus and the dorsum of the fifth metatarsal.

Charcot's joint. Joint enlargement with osteoarthritis caused by trophic disturbances in patients with tabes dorsalis, syringomyelia, and other neurologic disorders.

Chorea. Irregular and involuntary action of the muscles of the extremities and the face.

Chvostek's sign. A sign for tetany in which tapping the face in front of the ear produces spasm of the facial muscles.

Disconjugate deviation of eyes. Gaze palsy more severe at the medial rectus than at the lateral rectus, or vice versa.

Dissociated nystagmus. Nystagmus in which the movements of the two eyes are dissimilar.

Dysarthria. Imperfect pronunciation of words or phrases, causing them to be slurred together.

Dysdiadochokinesia. Difficulty in performing rapid alternating movement.

Dysmetria. Disturbances of the ability to measure distance and orientation in space while performing acts (especially with the eyes closed).

Dyssynergia. Loss of coordination in the performance of skilled or unskilled movements of the arms and legs.

Fasciculation. An uncoordinated contraction of skeletal muscle in which groups of muscle fibers innervated by the same neuron contract together.

Fibrillation. A local quivering of denervated muscle fibers usually not detectable by gross examination.

Foster Kennedy syndrome. Descending atrophy of one disc with papilledema of the other.

Foville's syndrome. Abducens palsy with homolateral facial and gaze palsy.

Gordon's sign. Plantar extension of the great toe when the calf muscles are squeezed firmly.

Graphesthesia. Ability to recognize numbers written on the skin.

Grasp reflex. Automatic clenching of the fist when an object is placed in the hand.

Hallpike's maneuver. A test performed with the patient initially seated on the edge of the examination table. The examiner turns the patient's head to the right while pulling the patient backward into a supine position with the patient's head hanging over the edge of the table. The test is repeated with the patient's head turned to the left. If one of these maneuvers produces nystagmus, the patient may have benign positional vertigo.

Hammer toe. A condition in which the proximal phalanx of the second toe is extremely extended and the two distal phalanges are flexed.

Hoffmann's sign. A test for overactive tendon reflexes in which the tapping of the nail of the index or middle finger causes flexion of the thumb.

Hoover's sign. A sign that differentiates between true and hysterical hemiplegia. In true hemiplegia, the patient thrusts the normal leg downward on attempting to raise the paralyzed leg. In hysterical hemiplegia, the patient attempts to raise the paralyzed leg without thrusting the normal leg downward.

Hysteria. A psychoneurotic disorder characterized by extreme emotionalism and involving disturbances of the psychic, somatic, and visceral functions.

Internuclear ophthalmoplegia. Gaze palsy that is more severe at the medial rectus than at the lateral rectus, or vice versa.

Kernig's sign. Inability to fully extend the leg when the thigh is flexed, a sign of meningeal irritation.

Kyphosis. Angular curvature of the spine; the convexity of the curvature is posterior.

Lasègue's sign. Extreme sensitivity to stretching the sciatic nerve trunk to less than 75 degrees on straight leg–raising test.

Lhermitte's sign. A sensation of an electric shock shooting into the extremities on flexion of the neck, occurring most typically in multiple sclerosis.

Marie-Foix sign. Forced dorsiflexion of the toes and withdrawal of the leg on transverse pressure of the tarsus.

Millard-Gubler syndrome. Abducens palsy with homolateral "peripheral" facial palsy and crossed hemiplegia.

Minor's sign. A method seen in patients with sciatica in which the patient rises to the standing position by leaning on the healthy side, bending the affected leg, and placing a hand on the back.

Myerson's sign. A sign of Parkinson's disease in which the eye blinks uncontrollably when an object is brought near it or when the brow is tapped.

Myotonic reflex. Sustained tonic contraction of a muscle on reflex stimulation; seen in myotonia dystrophica.

Nucleus. A group of neuron cell bodies in the central nervous system concerned with a particular function.

Nystagmus. An oscillatory movement of the eyeball.

Oppenheim sign. Plantar extension of the great toe in response to firm downward stroking of the medial border of the tibia.

Palm-to-chin reflex. Contraction of the homolateral mentalis muscles on stroking the palm, indicating pyramidal tract disease.

Parinaud's syndrome. Paralysis of the vertical gaze with disturbance of convergence caused by a lesion in the periaqueductal gray matter of the midbrain.

Patrick's sign. Hip pain on external rotation of the hip.

Past-pointing. A sign in which an attempt to bring the finger to a desired point results in the finger either falling short or passing beyond the right or left of the point.

Pes cavus. A form of clubfoot in which the arch is high.

Platybasia. A developmental deformity of the occipital bone and the upper cervical spine in which the foramen magnum is small and misshapen, the atlas is occipitalized, and the axis impinges on the brainstem.

Propulsion. A falling forward in walking (observed in paralysis agitans) in which the patient cannot stop at will.

Quadrantanopsia. Hemianopic defect delimited by the horizontal meridian.

Reaction of degeneration. Absence of the reaction of a muscle to faradic current and diminished response to a galvanic current.

Red-glass test. A test for the subclinical form of diplopia performed by placing a red glass before one eye, thus producing a false image. The patient with diplopia will see two images.

Retropulsion. Inability to stop running backward (observed in paralysis agitans).

Rinne test. A test to ascertain the ratio of air-to-bone conductivity performed by placing a vibrating tuning fork first to the mastoid process and then just adjacent to the ear (after the subject no longer hears the fork over the mastoid process). Normally, the air-to-bone ratio is 2:1. If the patient has sensorineural deafness, the ratio remains the same in the affected ear. If the patient has conductive deafness, the ratio becomes closer to 1:1.

Romberg's sign. Swaying to one side, forward, or backward when standing with the eyes closed and the feet close together.

Rossolimo's sign. Plantar flexion of the toes on stroking or tapping the plantar surface of the toes; occurs when there are lesions of the pyramidal tract.

Sacral sparing. Sparing of sensory loss in the distribution of the sacral nerves and the lower lumbar nerves in intramedullary lesions of the spinal cord.

Scoliosis. Lateral curvature of the spine.

Scotoma. A dark spot in the visual field.

Space-occupying lesion. A lesion, such as a tumor, abscess, hematoma, fracture, or herniated disc, that occupies space inside the skull or spinal column that is normally occupied by the components of the central nervous system.

Spasticity. An increased tonus or tension of a muscle that is associated with an exaggeration of the deep reflexes.

Spurling's test. Determines whether lateral flexion of the head produces pain or paresthesias in the upper extremity.

Steppage gait. The peculiar high-stepping gait seen in tabes dorsalis and certain peripheral neuropathies.

Tinel's sign. Paresthesias in the hand and fingers produced by tapping over the volar surface of the wrist or elbow.

Tomography. The technique of making roentgenograms of plane sections of solid objects.

Tract. A bundle of axonal fibers that perform a similar function.

Tromner's sign. Flexion of all four fingers and thumb on tapping of the volar aspect of the tip of the middle and index fingers while the fingers are partially flexed; indicates a pyramidal tract lesion.

Trousseau's sign. A sign for tetany in which carpal spasm can be elicited by compressing the upper arm.

Trunk ataxia. A disturbance of station and gait, with loss of balance and tendency to fall backward, caused by the lack of coordination between trunk movements and those of the extremities.

Two-point sensibility. Ability to discriminate one or two points placed apart at varying distances on the skin.

Wartenberg's leg-swinging test. Test in which the patient sits with the legs hanging freely; pendular swinging movements of the patient's legs produced by raising and suddenly releasing them are an indication of cerebellar disease.

Weber's syndrome. Paralysis of the oculomotor nerve on the side of the lesion and of the extremities and hypoglossal nerve on the opposite side.

Weber's test. A test for lateralization of auditory impairment, performed by placing a vibrating tuning fork on the vertex in the midline. If the patient has conductive hearing loss, he or she will hear the sound better on the side of the deafness. If the patient has sensorineural loss, the sound will be heard better on the side opposite the deafness.

Wernicke's hemianopic pupillary response. Lack of pupillary reaction to light from the "blind" side in hemianopsia.

Bibliography

Adler SN, Gasbarra DB, Adler-Klein D. *A pocket manual of differential diagnosis,* 4th ed. Philadelphia: Lippincott Williams & Wilkins, 2000.

Apierings Egilius LM. Advances in migraine treatment: the triptans. *Neurologist* 2001;7:113–121.

Brandt T, Von Kummer R, Muller-Kuppers M, et al. Thrombolytic therapy of acute basilar artery occlusion. Variables affecting recanalization and outcome. *Stroke* 1996;27:875–881.

Chestnut RM, Prough DS, eds. Critical care of severe head injury (symposium). *New Horiz* 1995;3:365–581.

Collins RD. *Algorithmic approach to treatment.* Baltimore: Williams & Wilkins, 1997.

Critchley EMR. *Neurological emergencies.* Philadelphia: WB Saunders, 1988.

Davis LE, Baldwin NG. Brian abscess. *Curr Treat Options Neurol* 1999;1:157–166.

Desai BT, Porter RJ, Penry JK. Psychogenic seizures. A study of 42 attacks in six patients with intensive monitoring. *Arch Neurol* 1982;39:202–209.

Devinsky O. Nonepileptic psychogenic seizures: quagmires of pathophysiology, diagnosis and treatment. *Epilepsia* 1998;39:458–462.

Dyck PJ, Lais AC, Ohta M, et al. Chronic inflammatory polyradiculoneuropathy. *Mayo Clin Proc.* 1975;50:621–637.

Ehrlich GE. Fibromyalgia: a virtual disease. *Clin Rheumatol* 2003;22:8–11.

Ehrlich GE. Pain is real: fibromyalgia isn't. *J Rheumatol* 2003;30:1666–1667.

Epstein O, Perkin GD, Cookson J, de Bono DP. *Pocket guide to clinical examination.* St. Louis: Mosby International, 1993.

Feske SK. Coma and confusional states: emergency diagnosis and management. *Neurol Clin* 1998;16:237–256.

Goldman L, Bennett JC. *Cecil textbook of medicine,* 21st ed. Philadelphia: WB Saunders, 2000.

Greenberg DA, Aminoff MJ, Simon RP. *Clinical neurology,* 5th ed. New York: Lange Medical Books, 2002.

Hart FD. *French's index of differential diagnosis,* 12th ed. Bristol: Wright, 1985.

Jacobs LD, Beck RW, Simon JH, et al. Intramuscular interferon beta-1a therapy initiated during a first demyelinating event in multiple sclerosis. *N Engl J Med* 2000;343:898–904.

Leis AA, Ross MA, Summers AK. Psychogenic seizures: ictal characteristics and diagnostic pitfalls. *Neurology* 1992;42:1848–1849.

Mesulam MM. Frontal cortex and behavior. *Ann Neurol* 1986;19:320–325.

Mulder DW, Kurland LT, Offord KP, Beard CM. Familial adult motor neuron disease: amyotrophic lateral sclerosis. *Neurology* 1986;36:511–517.

Nutt JG, Holford NHG. The response to levodopa in Parkinson's disease: imposing pharmacological law and order. *Ann Neurol* 1996;39:561–573.

O'Connor P. Diagnosis of central nervous system lupus. *Can J Neurol Sci* 1988;15:257–260.

Parkinson Study Group. Pramipexole vs. levodopa in treatment of Parkinson's disease. *JAMA* 2000;248:1931–1938.

Pourmand R. *Practicing neurology.* Boston: Butterworth Heinemann, 1999.

Rawson MD, Liversedge LA, Goldfarb G. Treatment of acute retrobulbar neuritis with corticotrophin. *Lancet* 1966;2:1044–1046.

Roos KL. Bacterial meningitis. *Curr Treat Options Neurol* 1999;1:147–156.

Rowland LP, ed. *Merritt's neurology,* 10th ed. Philadelphia: Lippincott Williams & Wilkins, 2000.

Samuels MA. The evaluation of comatose patients. *Hosp Pract* 1993;28:81–98.

Seller RH. *Differential diagnosis of common complaints,* 4th ed. Philadelphia: WB Saunders, 2000.

Strubb RL, Black FW. *The mental status examination in neurology,* 4th ed. Philadelphia: FA Davis, 1999.

Swann KW. *Management of severe head injury,* 2nd ed. New York: Aspen, 1988:166–167.

Vincent A, Palace J, Hilton-Jones D. Myasthenia gravis. *Lancet* 2001;357:2122–2128.

Whitely RJ. Viral encephalitis. *N Engl J Med* 1990;323:242–250.

INDEX

Note: Page numbers in *italics* indicate figures.